Practice rather than theory is the keynote of the *ABC of 1 to 7* in its straightforward advice on the diseases, emotional problems, and developmental disorders of early childhood. This has been amplified in this second edition which contains new chapters on recurrent headache and child abuse as well as extensive revisions of chapters on sleep problems, bronchial asthma, and primary and community care. The *ABC of 1 to 7* has become the standard guide for general practitioners, medical students, vocational trainees, and clinical medical officers. This second, revised and expanded edition brings it fully up to date.

ABC OF 1 TO 7

ABC OF 1 TO 7

H B VALMAN MD, FRCP

Consultant paediatrician,
Northwick Park Hospital and Clinical Research Centre,
Harrow, Middlesex

with contributions from
S K GOOLAMALI, J A FIXSEN, L PETER,
CLAIRE STURGE, MOYA TYSON, JUDITH WILSON

Articles published in
the *British Medical Journal*

Published by the British Medical Association
Tavistock Square, London WC1H 9JR

First edition 1982

Reprinted 1984

Second edition 1988

Reprinted 1989

Reprinted 1990

ISBN   0   7279   0104   4

Typeset in Great Britain by Latimer Trend & Company Ltd, Plymouth
Printed in Great Britain by The Universities Press (Belfast) Ltd.

Contents

Contents

TALKING TO CHILDREN

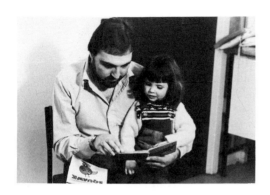

The newborn shares with lovers the ability to speak with the eyes. Communication develops from unintelligible sounds to gestures and finally words. An adult elicits these responses from a healthy child by normal speech or appropriate toys. Failure to respond may provide important evidence that there is a delay in development or a defect in the special senses. A quick response may help to distinguish between a child with a severe illness such as septicaemia or a child with a trivial problem who is just tired. Although guidelines on approaching children can be given, a normal range can be learnt only by attempting to communicate with every child.

In the consulting room

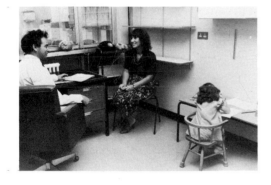

While the history is being taken from the mother the child will be listening and watching even if he appears preoccupied with play. If the doctor has formed a good rapport with the mother the child may talk easily when he is approached.

A small table and chair are needed at one side of the doctor's desk, and toys suitable for each age group should be scattered on this table, on the floor, and on adjacent shelves. The normal toddler will usually rush to this table and play. He remains quiet and while the history is being taken the doctor can observe the child's development of play, temperament, and dependence on his mother and the relationship between the parents and child. When the child is playing happily the doctor can wander over and start a conversation about the toys he has chosen. Even if the doctor knows a great deal about levels of communication and development the mother will display a child's abilities by talking to him herself. By observing her first, the doctor can pitch the method and type of communication at the right level. Ideally the eyes of the child and the doctor should be on the same horizontal plane so the doctor may have to sit on the floor, kneel, or crouch. Adequate time should be given to allow the child to respond, particularly those who cannot say words.

Questioning the child

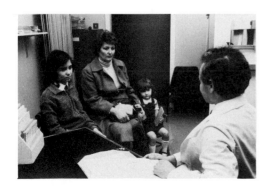

An older child may choose to sit next to the doctor and it may be possible to prompt him or her to give the history. The first words determine the success of the interview. The question "Where is the site of your abdominal pain, John?" will be greeted by silence. Questions which might start the conversation include "Which television programme do you like best?" "Did you come to the surgery by bus or car?" "What did you have for breakfast?" It may be necessary to make it clear to the mother that the doctor wants to hear what the child has to say. She may interpose answers because she can give a more accurate history, wants to avert criticism, is overprotective, or wants to save the doctor's time. Ideally, the child and his parents should be seen together and later separately, but a child who does not speak freely in the presence of his parents is unlikely, during the first visit, to speak more openly when he is separated.

Talking to children

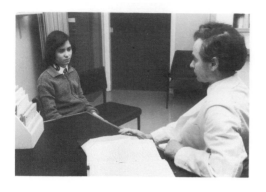

The child should be addressed by his own name or the nickname that he likes. A little flattery sometimes helps—for example, admiring a girl's dress or saying that a toddler is grown up. A cheeky smile in response to a question as to whether a boy fights with his sister shows that you are on the right wavelength. For children who are not yet talking it may be possible to play a simple game of putting things into a cup and taking them out or making scribbles on a piece of paper alternately with the child. Simple words should be used which the child is likely to understand, but if a doctor uses a childish word when the patient knows it by a normal word he will think that the doctor is treating him as a baby and underestimating his abilities.

Reassuring mother and child

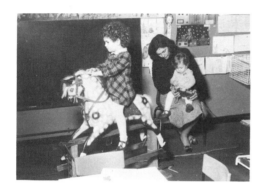

Whatever the age, talking to the child while examining him has several advantages. If the doctor says, "That's good" after listening to the heart for a long time this reassures the mother that he has found nothing dreadful. Saying to the child, "You are very good this time" or "You are very grown up" often keeps the child still while his ears are being examined or his abdomen palpated. Even if the child does not understand the meaning of the words, the tone of the examiner's voice may calm him and allow prolonged detailed examination without protest.

Going to the doctor should be a treat, so more exciting books, toys, and equipment should be available than are present at home. In the past many doctors used sweets to soften the trauma of a visit to the surgery but many mothers now frown on doctors who have apparently not heard the advice of dentists. A sweet in the mouth of the child during examination of the throat can be dangerous. A properly equipped waiting room and consulting room will enable a more accurate clinical diagnosis to be made and provides an incentive for the child to come again and not to want to go home on the first visit.

THE TERRIBLE 2s

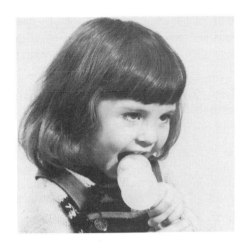

The period between 2 and 3 years may bring disillusion to parents. Their idealised innocent angel seems to have become a calculating devil. Until then the words "mischievous," "naughty," "little devil" were terms of endearment. At 2 years they become accurate terms of description: the child's behaviour appears to be planned to cause the maximum anguish.

Independence versus dependence

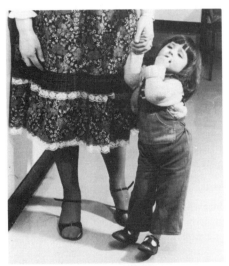

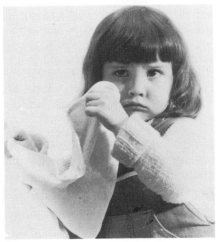

At about the age of 2 the child discovers that he can control what happens around him when he begins to talk and can decide when to pass urine or stools. A conflict develops between his desire to assert his independence and his wish to regress to an earlier stage of dependence. The independence may be expressed in the defiance of temper tantrums, but increasing independence brings a fear of insecurity, which may be expressed as a phobia, overdependence on items that represent security—for example, a blanket—and rocking. The conflict between independence and security is seen in lapses of sphincter control and in feeding and speech problems.

At the age of 2 symbolic thought is just beginning but it is self-centred. The high level of understanding and speech combined with a disregard for the needs of others may lead the parents to think that their child wants to hurt them. A mother might be trying to dress a 2 year old quickly to be on time for an appointment, but he treats the whole event as a game, running and hiding, and does not understand why his mother loses her temper. These episodes also illustrate the toddler's inability to see any behaviour from the other person's point of view. A violent temper tantrum, even when he kicks or bites his mother, is related to what the child can achieve from the action and is not motivated by a desire to inflict pain.

At this age there is also little sense of time and if the mother goes next door to see a neighbour for a few minutes the child may fear that he has been abandoned for ever.

The terrible 2s

Effects on parents

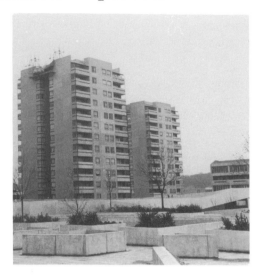

The other half of the picture of the terrible 2 year old is the distraught parents, particularly the mother. Mothers often feel that they cannot cope and become depressed and anxious. Their families, friends, and husbands may support them, but living in high-rise flats may have an adverse effect. The referral rate for 2–3 year olds to family doctors is the highest of any age group, including the elderly. The consultations are usually ostensibly about coughs and colds, but the real reason may be that the mother is having great difficulty in coping at all. Accurate diagnosis and sound advice at this stage can be an important part of preventive child health. Two years is also a common age gap between children, so the mother may be pregnant or just have had another baby. The toddler may show resentment, sometimes very intense, towards the new baby, and the parents feel hurt by this resentment. These negative feelings may precipitate or accentuate any of the problems seen in this age group, and the parents' disillusion may lead to feelings of guilt or doubt about where they went wrong in bringing up their child. These responses may reinforce the confusion of feelings in the child and worsen the problems.

Intervention

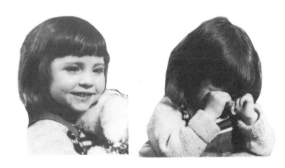

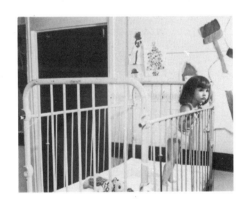

Every baby is born with a different temperament and while the parents may be genetically responsible there is nothing they can do to change it. Children vary in their moodiness, response to frustration, and adaptability. They also vary in the intervals between micturition and defecation and their need for sleep and food. The "easiest" child temperamentally is a child who is not very intense or moody, has a high threshold for frustration, is not particularly active, and adapts easily. Such a child may not present any particular problems at 2. The converse describes a "difficult" child. If this variability is explained to the parents it may improve their understanding of their child, remove some of their guilt, and enable them to handle the child better.

Intervention is effective only if the parents can see the child's problem in perspective and are more concerned with resolving it than with concentrating on the feeling the child's behaviour arouses in them. Many of the problems 2 year olds pose are habit problems—for example, sleep problems—and the habits have developed because the parents have reinforced them in some way. Despite the parents' bitter complaints about their child's behaviour they are often unable to change their own behaviour. For example, if a 2 year old who has frequent temper tantrums makes his mother feel that she is responsible for his not being happy and she thinks that the tantrums are a sign of insecurity she will not be firm with the child and will not follow the doctor's advice. Families often claim to have tried everything when in fact they have tried no one method with commitment. They may see any intervention as cruel and unloving. If the mother realises that she, the child, and the family would have an easier time if there were fewer tantrums she can be advised to ignore them. She must ignore them every time and if necessary leave the child alone in the room or put him in another one. When the child is finally calm, however long this takes, she should then behave normally and accept the child fully: she should never give additional treats in the form of sweets or cuddles. Behavioural studies show that if a subject finds that he can ever "get away" with a particular form of behaviour he will repeatedly try it out because he knows exceptions to the new, firm response are possible. The parents need to know that any inconsistency will lead to failure. When the child realises that both parents have an agreed pattern of attitudes his temper tantrums will stop.

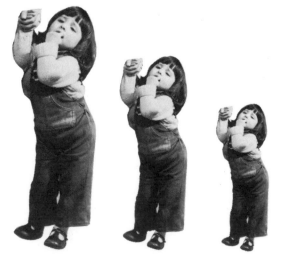

Sleeping and eating

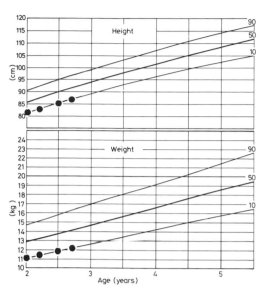

The approach to sleeping and eating problems is similar. Healthy toddlers gain weight normally in spite of their mother's protests that they eat very little. They seem to know instinctively their minimum requirements. Refusal to eat is a very powerful weapon as it challenges the mother's ability to nurture her child. If the mother is reassured that the child will not harm himself by not eating then she will not press him when he refuses.

Toilet training may be tackled either by highly structured training schemes or by waiting and attempting training after an interval. Most 2 year old children have problems with bladder and bowel control at some time, but in most they resolve spontaneously at the age of 3 or 4.

Problems of dependence

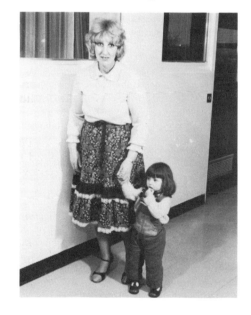

Problems relating to dependence, such as fears and phobias, excessive use of security items, or excessive masturbation or nightmares need a very different approach and it is the parents who need most help in understanding the problems and helping the child. They need to learn not to reinforce the anxieties by over-reacting to the child's fear but to help the child learn to feel in control of his situation and more confident. Encouraging the child to play or act out things he worries about may help. Separation fears are a common anxiety, even when there seems no real reason for them. Difficulty in separation at this age is normal and should never be seen as a problem. If, however, a 2 year old can learn to separate from his mother and trust her to return he will become more confident and less vulnerable.

Better by 3

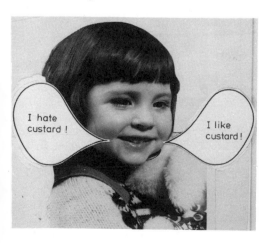

I hate custard!

I like custard!

All the problems that have been discussed are variations in behaviour that fall within a normal range. When doctors are consulted they should be prepared to find that they cannot help because the family does not want to change the way it behaves, in which case reassurance that the child's behaviour will probably improve with time may be all that is possible. As the child approaches the age of 3 years he becomes more sociable and learns to share and to take turns. Whether the family is receptive or resistant to suggestions of help, an explanation of why the child behaves as he does may be valuable and help to make the parents feel understood.

In some cases the child may need to be referred for specialist help. Those with speech problems, for example, should see a paediatrician or speech therapist. If the child's behaviour or the family's reaction is well outside the normal range then he should be referred to a child psychiatrist, and if the whole family is disrupted by the child's behaviour the help of the social services department may be needed.

SLEEP PROBLEMS

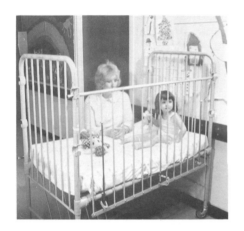

Some children will not sleep when they are put to bed, but the most distressing problem for parents is those who keep waking in the night or wake in the early morning. The mother rapidly becomes exhausted, and marital discord may follow while the child remains fresh. Sleep problems are common. Twenty per cent of infants wake early or in the night at the age of 2, and it is still a problem in 10% at 4½. Between these ages the symptoms resolve in some children but appear for the first time in others. Drugs may cause irritability and sleep problems—for instance, theophylline preparations for bronchial asthma or phenobarbitone for febrile convulsions.

Normal patterns

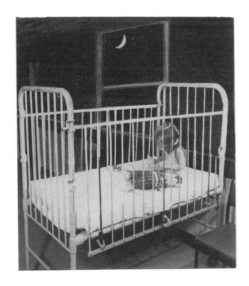

During the first few weeks of life some babies sleep almost continuously for the 24 hours whereas others sleep for only about 12 hours. This pattern of needing little sleep may persist so that by the age of 1 year an infant may wake regularly at 2 am and remain awake for two hours or more. As these infants approach the age of 3 they tend to wake at 6 am and then remain awake for the rest of the day. Many 2-year-old children sleep for an hour or two in the afternoons, and some have a similar amount of sleep in the mornings as well. A child who spends four hours of the day sleeping may spend four hours of the night awake. Parents often worry that an infant is suffering from lack of sleep and wrongly ascribe his poor appetite or frequent colds to this cause.

During the night babies and children often wake up, open their eyes, lift their heads, and move their limbs. If they are not touched most of them fall back to sleep again. A mother who wakes as a result of this moving, gets out of bed, and looks at her child may keep him awake. If this happens several times every night it may prevent the infant from developing normal patterns of sleep

History

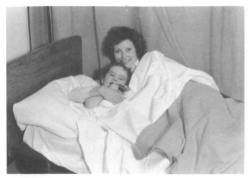

The doctor needs to take a full history. He needs details of the sleep pattern, when the problem began, and measures taken to resolve it. It should be possible to determine whether the child has always needed little sleep or whether he has developed a habit of crying in order to get into his parents' comfortable bed. He should also explore the reason why the mother has sought advice at this stage. She should be asked about any change in the house, where the child sleeps, whether he attends a playgroup, and who looks after him during the day. Illnesses in the child or family and marital and social backgrounds also need considering. A physical examination usually shows no abnormality, but occasionally there may be signs of acute otitis media.

Difficulty in going to sleep

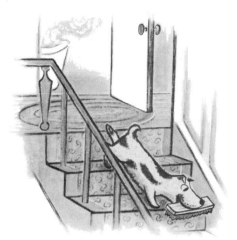

Harry was a white dog with black spots
who liked everything,
except... having a bath.
So one day when he heard the water
running in the tub,
he took the scrubbing brush...

Difficulty in getting to sleep can often be avoided by starting a bedtime ritual in infancy. A warm bath followed by being wrapped in particular blankets may later be replaced by the mother or father reading from a book or singing nursery rhymes before the light is turned out. Some children have been frightened by a nightmare and fear going to sleep in case it is repeated. A small night light or a light on the landing showing through the open door may allay this fear. A soft cuddly toy of any type can lie next to the infant from shortly after birth, and seeing this familiar toy again may help to induce sleep.

The mother should be told that during the night babies often open their eyes and move their limbs and heads. She should be asked to resist getting up to see the baby as the noise of getting out of bed may wake him and he may then remain awake. If he does wake he may be pacified with a drink and may then fall asleep. His drink is to provide comfort rather than to assuage any thirst.

Parents whose young children sleep a great deal during the day can discourage them from doing this by taking them out shopping or giving them other diversions, and they may then sleep well at night.

Sleep disturbance is a common reaction to the trauma of admission to hospital or moving house, and taking the child into the parent's room for a few weeks may help to reassure the child that he has not been abandoned. If there are toys or other things to amuse them some children who wake in the night will play for hours, talking to themselves and not crying. Parents need to be reassured that this is perfectly normal and that they are lucky that the child does not demand their attention.

If the child is prepared to go to sleep at a certain time but the parents would like to advance it by an hour they can put him to bed five minutes earlier each night until the planned bedtime is achieved.

Behaviour modification and drugs

Mon	Sleep	Nap.	Sleep

Shade in the times your child is asleep ▨ Leave blank the times your child is awake

Midnight   Noon   Midnight
12.00 2.00 4.00 6.00 8.00 10.00 12.00 2.00 4.00 6.00 8.00 10.00 12.00

Mon													
Tue													
Wed													
Thur													
Fri													
Sat													
Sun													

Day	Time to bed	Time to sleep	First problem	What did you do ?	Second problem	What did you do ?	Time woke up in morning
Mon							
Tue							
Wed							
Thur							
Fri							
Sat							
Sun							

When the child wakes frequently during the night and cries persistently until he is taken into his parents' bed a plan of action is needed. If there is an obvious cause, such as acute illness, recent admission to hospital, or a new baby, the problem may resolve itself within a few weeks, and at first there need be no change in management. If there is no obvious cause the parents are asked to keep a record of the child's sleep pattern for two weeks (see sleep history chart). This helps to determine where the main problem lies and can be used as a comparison with treatment.

Both parents are seen at the next visit; both need to accept that they must be firm and follow the plan exactly. Behaviour modification is the only method that produces long-term improvement, but it can be combined with drugs initially if the mother is at breaking point.

Behaviour modification separates the mother from the child gradually or abruptly, depending on the parents' and doctor's philosophy. The slow method starts with the mother giving a drink and staying with the child for decreasing lengths of time. In the next stage no drink is given. Then she speaks to the child through the closed door and, finally, does not go to him at all. The abrupt method consists of letting the child cry it out; he stops after three or four nights. There are an infinite number of variations between these extremes, and the

Sleep problems

| | | If your child is still crying | | |
Day	At first episode	Second episode	Third episode	Subsequent episodes
1	5	10	15	15
2	10	15	20	20
3	15	20	25	25
4	20	25	30	30
5	25	30	35	35

Number of minutes to wait before going into your child briefly

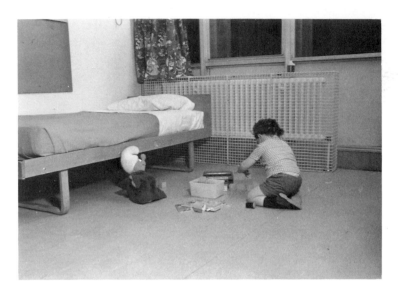

temperament of the parents, child, and doctor will determine what is acceptable.

Another approach is to increase the waiting time before going to the child. In severe cases a written programme of several small changes can be given to the mother and she can be seen again by the health visitor or family doctor after each step has been achieved. The mother will need to be reassured that the child will not develop a hernia from crying or vomit or choke, and neighbours may be pacified by being told that the child will soon be cured.

Many sleep problems can be resolved without drugs, but some mothers are so exhausted by loss of sleep that they cannot manage a programme of behaviour modification unless the infant receives some preliminary sedation. The most satisfactory drug in this age group is trimeprazine tartrate, 3 mg/kg body weight given one hour before going to bed. These large doses are needed as lower, more conventional doses are usually ineffective. The full dose is given for two weeks, followed by a half dose for a week; the drug is then given on alternate nights for a week. The objective is to change the pattern of sleeping. A behaviour modification plan is needed during the third and subsequent weeks.

Children around the age of 2 who wake early in the morning may be helped by giving them a low divan bed instead of a cot. They can get out of bed and play with their toys on the floor and leave the rest of the household to sleep.

RESPIRATORY TRACT INFECTION

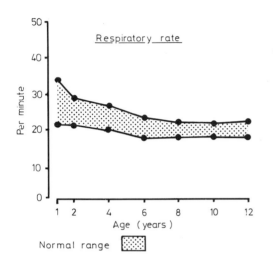

Respiratory rate

Per minute

Age (years)

Normal range

Infection of the respiratory tract is a common cause of illness in children. Although pathogens are often not confined to anatomical boundaries, the infections may be classified as:

(a) upper respiratory tract—common cold, tonsillitis and pharyngitis, and acute otitis media;

(b) middle respiratory tract—acute laryngitis and epiglottitis;

(c) lower respiratory tract—bronchitis, bronchopneumonia, and segmental pneumonia.

Viruses, which cause most respiratory tract infections, and bacterial infections produce similar clinical illnesses. Different viruses may produce an identical picture, or the same virus may cause different clinical syndromes. Clinically it may not be possible to determine whether the infection is due to viruses, bacteria, or both. If the infection is suspected of being bacterial it is safest to prescribe an antibiotic, as the results of virus studies are often received after the acute symptoms have passed. The commonest bacterial pathogens are pneumococci. Less common are *Haemophilus influenzae*, group A β-haemolytic streptococci, *Staphylococcus aureus*, group B β-haemolytic streptococci, Gram-negative bacteria, and anaerobic bacteria.

Common cold (coryza)

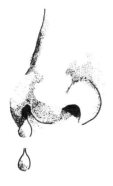

Preschool children usually have about six colds each year. The main symptoms are sneezing, nasal discharge, and mild fever. Similar symptoms may occur in the early phases of infection with rotavirus and be followed by vomiting and diarrhoea. Postnasal discharge may produce coughing. The commonest complication is acute otitis media, but secondary bacterial infection of the lower respiratory tract sometimes occurs.

There is no specific treatment for the common cold, and antibiotics should not be given. A danger with nasal drops is that they will run down into the lower respiratory tract and carry the infection there.

Acute bronchitis

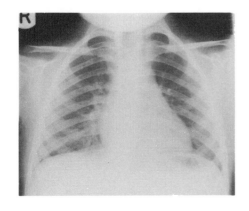

Acute bronchitis often follows a viral upper respiratory tract infection and there is always a cough, which may be accompanied by wheezing. There is no fever. The respiratory rate is normal and the symptoms resolve within a week. The only signs, which are not constantly present, are rhonchi. Since it is usually due to a virus, antibiotics are indicated only if the illness is severe or a bacterial cause is shown.

Respiratory tract infection

Recurrent bronchitis

Recurrent bronchitis

?

Bronchial asthma

Two separate episodes of acute bronchitis may occur in a normal child in a year. If attacks are more frequent at any age bronchial asthma should be considered (see page 17). Viruses cause the majority of attacks of bronchitis and will precipitate most attacks of bronchial asthma. The symptoms and signs of both conditions are similar, but recurrent symptoms suggest bronchial asthma. The diagnosis of bronchial asthma is important because a range of treatments is available.

If there is a persistent or recurrent cough a chest radiograph should be performed to exclude persistent segmental or lobar collapse. A Mantoux test for tuberculosis should be performed, a sweat test to exclude cystic fibrosis, and plasma immunoglobulin studies to exclude rare syndromes.

Bronchopneumonia and segmental pneumonia

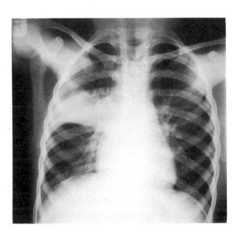

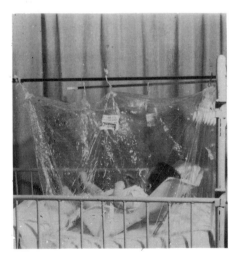

Pneumonia is acute inflammation of the lung alveoli. In bronchopneumonia the infection is spread throughout the bronchial tree whereas in segmental pneumonia it is confined to the alveoli in one segment or lobe. A raised respiratory rate at rest distinguishes pneumonia from bronchitis. Cough, fever, and flaring of the alae nasi are usually present and there may be reduced breath sounds over the affected area as well as crepitations. A chest radiograph, which is needed in every child with suspected pneumonia, may show extensive changes when there are no localising signs in the chest. The radiograph may show an opacity confined to a single segment or lobe but there may be bilateral patchy changes. Bacterial cultures of throat swabs and blood should be performed before treatment is started. Ideally virological studies of nasopharyngeal secretions and estimations of virus antibody titres in sera collected in the acute and convalescent phases should also be done.

Children with pneumonia are best treated in hospital as they often need oxygen treatment. Antibiotics should be prescribed for all cases of pneumonia, although later a viral cause may be discovered. Ampicillin and flucloxacillin are given intravenously by bolus injection for bronchopneumonia, whereas penicillin, ampicillin, or amoxycillin can be used in segmental pneumonia as the pneumococcus is the commonest pathogen. Severely ill children may have either staphylococcal pneumonia or a Gram-negative infection and they need an additional antibiotic. Fusidic acid is added for suspected staphylococcal infection and gentamicin for Gram-negative infection. Oral erythromycin may be given to patients who are sensitive to penicillins and to those whose failure to respond to the other antibiotics suggest that they have mycoplasma or chlamydia infection. Antibiotic treatment can be modified when the results of bacterial cultures are available. Intravenous fluids may be needed and oxygen treatment is best provided in a tent.

The chest radiograph of a child with segmental or lobar pneumonia should be repeated after one month.

TONSILLITIS AND OTITIS MEDIA

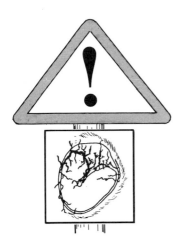

Upper respiratory tract infections become more common after the age of 1 year. In the child the pharynx, tonsils, and middle ear are close together and it may seem arbitrary to divide them anatomically and prescribe separate treatment for each area. Although failing to give specific treatment for acute tonsillitis rarely results in sequelae, lack of treatment of acute otitis media may lead to bursting of the drum and a chronic discharge. As preschool children have about six upper respiratory tract infections each year, these problems are extremely common.

Tonsillitis and pharyngitis

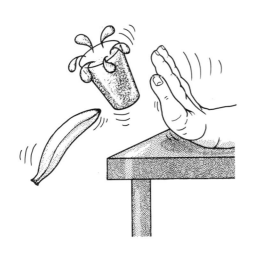

Sunday	Monday	Tuesday	Wednesday	Thursday
✗	✗	✗	✗	✗
Friday	**Saturday**	PENICILLIN	**Monday**	**Tuesday**
✗	7	8	9	10

In children aged under 3 years the commonest presenting features of tonsillitis are fever and refusal to eat, but a febrile convulsion may occur at the onset. Older children may complain of a sore throat or enlarged cervical lymph nodes, which may or may not be painful. Viral and bacterial causes cannot be distinguished clinically since a purulent follicular exudate may be present in both. Ideally a throat swab should be sent to the laboratory before starting treatment to determine a bacterial cause for the symptoms and to help to indicate the pathogens currently in the community. If there has been a recurrence of group A haemolytic streptococci in outbreaks of sore throat, a more liberal use of penicillin is justified during this period. As this organism is the only important bacterium causing tonsillitis, penicillin is the drug of choice and the only justification for using another antibiotic is a convincing history of hypersensitivity to penicillin. In that case the alternatives are erythromycin or co-trimoxazole. In the absence of an outbreak of group A streptococcus infection the indication for oral penicillin is fever or severe systemic symptoms. The drug should be continued for at least 10 days if a streptococcal infection is confirmed. Parents often stop the drug after a few days as the symptoms have often abated and the medicine is unpalatable. The organism is not eradicated unless a full 10-day course is given.

Viral infections often produce two peaks on the temperature chart.

An extensive thick white shaggy exudate on the tonsils (sometimes invading the pharynx) suggests infectious mononucleosis, and a full blood count, examination of the blood film, and a Monospot test are indicated. A membranous exudate on the tonsils suggests diphtheria and an urgent expert opinion should be sought.

Fluids can be given while there is dysphagia, and regular paracetamol during the first 24 to 48 hours reduces fever and discomfort.

A peritonsillar abscess (quinsy) is now extremely rare. It displaces the tonsil medially so that the swollen soft palate obscures the tonsil and the uvula is displaced across the midline. The advice of an ENT surgeon is needed urgently.

Tonsillitis and otitis media

Acute otitis media

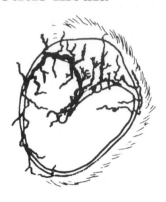

Ampicillin
Amoxycillin
Co-trimoxazole

Erythromycin
Cephalexin

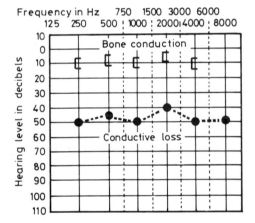

AMPLIVOX AUDIOGRAM

Secretory otitis media

Routine hearing test

After acute otitis media

Behaviour problem

Slow learning

"Switching off"

Pain is the main symptom of acute otitis media and is one of the reasons why a child wakes crying in the night. If the otitis media is bilateral the child has difficulty in locating the site of the pain. The pain is relieved if the drum ruptures. Viruses probably cause over half the cases of acute otitis media, but a viral or bacterial origin cannot be distinguished clinically. The commonest bacteria are pneumococci, group A haemolytic streptococci, and *Haemophilus influenzae*.

Children are often fascinated by the light of the auriscope, and the auriscope speculum can be placed on a doll's ear or the child's forearm to reassure him. Gentleness is essential and the speculum should never be pushed too far into the external meatus because this causes discomfort. If the pinna is pulled gently outwards to open the meatal canal the tympanic membrane is visible with the tip of a speculum only as far as the outer end of the meatus. In early cases of otitis media there are dilated vessels on the upper and posterior part of the drum. Later the tympanic membrane becomes congested and bulging and the light reflex becomes less clear. In severe cases of otitis media there may be bullous formation on the drum. This may cause acute pain initially, is not associated with a particular organism, and calls for no treatment apart from that of the acute otitis media. Swelling or tenderness behind the pinna should always be sought as mastoiditis may be easily missed.

The choice of initial treatment lies between ampicillin, amoxycillin, and co-trimoxazole. If there is no improvement in the drum after two or three days another antibiotic should be substituted. Erythromycin and cephalexin are second-line drugs. There is no evidence that any form of ear drops are helpful in acute otitis media with an intact drum. Antibiotics should be given for 10 days and the ears examined again before the course is stopped. Ideally a hearing test should be performed three months after each attack of acute otitis media to detect residual deafness and secretory otitis media (glue ear). One study showed that, after the first attack of acute otitis media in infants, which was treated with antimicrobial agents, 40% had no middle ear effusion after one month and 90% after three months.

If three attacks of acute otitis media occur within three months and the drum has a normal appearance between attacks, a prophylactic drug should be considered. The most suitable drug is co-trimoxazole given at half the standard 24-hour dose in the evening only. This treatment is given for three months, and several studies have shown that the incidence of further attacks is reduced during that period. If the appearance of the drums does not return to normal after a 10-day course of treatment for acute otitis media the possibility of secretory otitis media should be considered.

Secretory otitis media may be discovered during a routine hearing test. It may be found as a result of impaired hearing shown after an attack of acute otitis media. The insidious onset of this problem may result in the child presenting at school with a behaviour problem, slow learning, or periods of "switching off" during lessons, which may be misinterpreted as petit mal. Hearing may fluctuate; some weeks it may be normal but severely impaired at other times. Routine screening tests may be performed during the good period and produce a false sense of security.

Fluid, often of glue-like consistency, fills the middle ear cavity in glue ear. This fluid reduces the movements of the tympanic membrane, resulting in hearing impairment. The cause is unknown, but it has been suggested that the middle ear fluid is unable to drain along the Eustachian tube into the nasopharynx due to obstruction of the tube by mucopus or oedema.

The tympanic membrane may show a variety of abnormalities. There may be dilated vessels along the handle of the malleus and round the periphery of the drum, and they may radiate over the surface. The membrane may be normal in colour, pale amber, slate, or dark blue depending on the nature of the middle ear fluid.

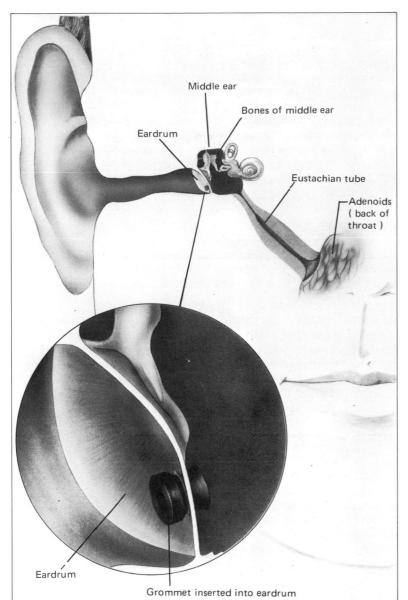

Middle ear

Bones of middle ear

Eardrum

Eustachian tube

Adenoids
(back of
throat)

Eardrum

Grommet inserted into eardrum

If secretory otitis media is suspected the child should be seen by an ear, nose, and throat surgeon. After the clinical examination a hearing test and impedance audiometry are performed. This test measures the movements of the drum by a special probe in the external auditory meatus. If the results of the impedance audiometry test is abnormal it must be repeated after six weeks or three months as a single observation is unreliable. He usually waits 3 months in the hope that the effusion will diminish or resolve. Previously, oral antihistamines and decongestant nose drops were given to improve Eustachian tube drainage. Recent studies have shown that oral antihistamines have no clinical value and there is no evidence that nose drops are effective. If the effusion persists myringotomy is performed under general anaesthesia. The effusion is aspirated and a grommet may be inserted through the incision. This allows air into the middle ear, a role eventually resumed by the Eustachian tube. The insertion of grommets is avoided unless there is good evidence that the duration of the effusion has been long. Grommets may cause scarring of the drum and the long-term effects of this complication are not known.

The grommet usually becomes blocked about six to nine months after insertion. It is gradually extruded and falls out between two months and two years after insertion. The incision heals spontaneously. Glue ear sometimes recurs and the grommet may need to be inserted several times. Swimming should be avoided while the grommet is in place. The value of adenoidectomy is controversial.

By the age of 7 or 8 years children who have had secretory otitis media usually have normal ears and normal hearing. This occurs as part of the natural history of the problem and is not related to the treatment. This means that provided the child with secretory otitis media has adequate hearing for his education no medical or surgical treatment is needed. Apart from pure tone audiometry discussed above, the best test of adequate hearing is the level of speech development, and if significant hearing loss is detected or suspected speech should be assessed and monitored regularly by a speech therapist. A child with secretory otitis media may have another factor, such as intellectual impairment or social deprivation, as the main cause of the delay in his speech development.

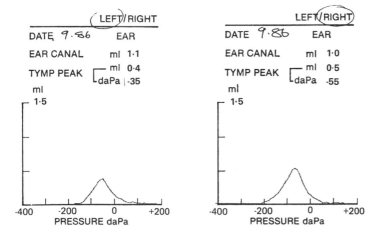

	LEFT/RIGHT	
DATE 9.86	EAR	
EAR CANAL	ml	1·1
TYMP PEAK	ml	0·4
ml	daPa	-35

	LEFT/RIGHT	
DATE 9.86	EAR	
EAR CANAL	ml	1·0
TYMP PEAK	ml	0·5
ml	daPa	-55

1·5

-400   -200   0   +200
PRESSURE daPa

1·5

-400   -200   0   +200
PRESSURE daPa

Impedance audiometry showing movements of the tympanic membrane in response to changes in pressure in the auditory canal

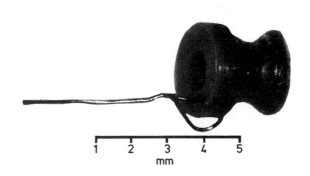

1   2   3   4   5
mm

Tonsillitis and otitis media

Indications for tonsillectomy

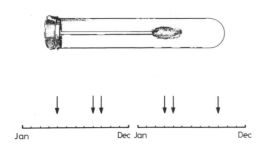

If bacterial infection of the tonsils is suspected because there is pus on the tonsils and if group A haemolytic streptococci are grown from swabs more than three times a year in two consecutive years, tonsillectomy may be indicated. Many paediatricians would consider that these criteria are not stringent enough, though tonsillectomy would be a rare operation even if these less stringent criteria were followed. An absolute indication for tonsillectomy is such gross enlargement of the tonsils that they meet in the midline between attacks of infection and cause stridor or apnoea. Another indication is recurrent febrile convulsions associated with attacks of definite follicular tonsillitis.

Indications for adenoidectomy

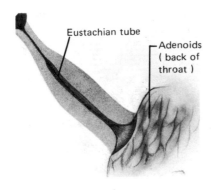

Children with more than three episodes of acute otitis media a year or those with secretory otitis media (glue ear) should be seen by an ENT surgeon. As well as aspiration of the middle ear and the insertion of a grommet, adenoidectomy is usually considered. If the surgeon considers that adenoidal tissue encroaches on the nasopharyngeal orifice of the Eustachian tube he may perform an adenoidectomy. Partial nasal obstruction causing snoring at night and mouth breathing during the day with recurrent sore throat may be an indication for adenoidectomy, although there is a high rate of spontaneous cure if the parents can be persuaded to wait.

STRIDOR

Stridor is noisy breathing caused by obstruction in the pharynx, larynx, or trachea. It may be distinguished from partial obstruction of the bronchi by the absence of rhonchi. Although most cases are due to acute laryngitis and may resolve with the minimum of care, similar features are found in acute epiglottitis and may cause sudden death. Stridor is recognised as one of the most ominous signs in childhood. Any doctor should be able to recognise the sound over the telephone and arrange to see the child immediately. Examination of the throat may precipitate total obstruction of the airway and should be attempted only in the presence of an anaesthetist and facilities for intubation.

Laryngitis

Epiglottitis

Foreign body

History and management

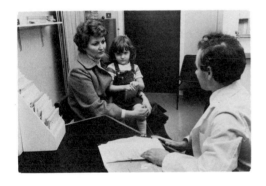

A glance at the child will show whether urgent treatment is needed or whether there is time for a detailed history to be taken. The doctor needs to know when the symptoms started and whether there is nasal discharge or cough. Choking over food, especially peanuts, or the abrupt onset of symptoms after playing alone with small objects suggests that a foreign body is present.

During the taking of the history and the examination the mother should remain near her child and be encouraged to hold him and to talk to him. All unpleasant procedures such as venepuncture should be avoided. This reduces the possibility of struggling, which may precipitate complete airway obstruction. Agitation and struggling raise the peak flow rate and move secretions, which results in increased hypoxia and the production of more secretions.

Acute laryngotracheitis

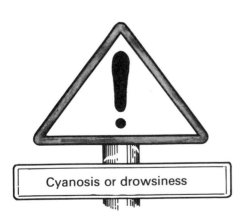

Cyanosis or drowsiness

Acute laryngitis causes partial obstruction of the larynx. It is characterised by inspiratory and expiratory stridor (noisy breathing), cough, and hoarseness. The laryngeal obstruction is due to oedema, spasm, and secretions. Affected children are usually aged 6 months to 3 years, and the symptoms are most severe in the early hours of the morning. Recession of the intercostal spaces indicates significant obstruction and cyanosis or drowsiness shows that total obstruction of the airway is imminent.

Complete airway obstruction may occur during examination of the throat of a child with stridor. The examination should be attempted only in the presence of an anaesthetist and facilities for intubation, preferably in the anaesthetic room of the operating theatre.

A child often improves considerably after inhaling steam, which is provided easily by turning on the hot taps in the bathroom. Mild cases may be treated successfully at home using this method but the child must be visited every few hours to determine whether he is deteriorating and needs to be admitted to hospital. Continuous stridor or recession demands urgent hospital admission. Oxygen with increased humidity can be given with a special humidifier by nursing the child in a small tent (croupette), but it is difficult to observe the child and he cannot see his parents. These disadvantages can be avoided by using a large humidifier without a tent, but it may not be so effective. Hypoxaemia or thirst may cause restlessness and should

Stridor

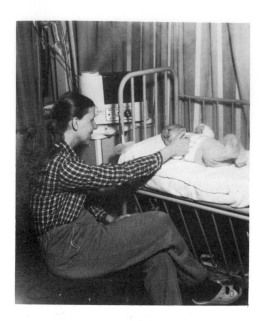

be corrected and sedatives avoided. Rarely the obstruction needs to be relieved by passing an endotracheal tube or performing a tracheostomy.

Acute laryngotracheitis is usually caused by a viral infection and therefore infants with mild symptoms do not need antibiotics. In a few cases *Staphylococcus aureus* or *Haemophilus influenzae* is present and the associated septicaemia makes the child appear very ill. Bacterial infection is characterised by plaques of debris and pus on the surface of the trachea, partially obstructing it, just below the vocal cords. If bacterial infection is suspected flucloxacillin and ampicillin are given intravenously. Acute epiglottitis and acute laryngitis may be indistinguishable clinically since stridor and progressive upper airway obstruction are the main features of both. Some authorities prefer to give ampicillin to all infants with the characteristic symptoms. Some paediatricians give steroids as well. The dose of hydrocortisone is 100 mg intramuscularly or intravenously repeated once after two hours. No effect is seen for at least two hours. Later betamethasone should be given at a dose of 3 mg intravenously every six hours but only until signs of improvement appear. Children with severe symptoms should be managed in the intensive care unit.

Acute epiglottitis

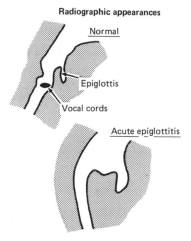

Radiographic appearances

Normal

Epiglottis

Vocal cords

Acute epiglottitis

Children with epiglottitis are usually aged over 2 years; drooling and dysphagia are common, and the child usually wants to sit upright. When the obstruction is very severe the stridor becomes ominously quieter. There is usually an associated septicaemia with *Haemophilus influenzae*.

If epiglottitis is suspected the child should be transferred urgently to hospital. Facilities for intubation or tracheostomy must be available when the throat is examined because the examination may cause complete airway obstruction. The epiglottis is red and swollen. Acute epiglottitis has a high mortality. Some units have found a lateral radiograph of the neck helpful in distinguishing between acute laryngitis and acute epiglottitis. The films must be taken in the intensive care unit with the child in the upright position in the presence of a doctor skilled in intubation. Since it is impossible to distinguish clinically between infection with *H influenzae* and a viral infection intravenous chloramphenicol should be given.

Other causes and emergency management of foreign bodies

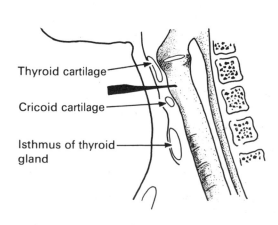

Thyroid cartilage

Cricoid cartilage

Isthmus of thyroid gland

Even if the symptoms have settled and there are no abnormal signs, a history of the onset of sudden choking or coughing can never be ignored. A radiograph of the neck and chest should be taken and may show a hypertranslucent lung on the side of a foreign body, a shift of the mediastinum, or, less commonly, collapse of part of the lung or a radio-opaque foreign body. The radiograph may be considered normal. Bronchoscopy may be needed to exclude a foreign body even if the chest radiograph appears to be normal. Stridor in a child who has had scalds or burns or has inhaled steam from a kettle suggests that intubation or tracheostomy may be needed urgently.

If the cause of stridor is likely to be a foreign body below the larynx the object should be removed immediately by a thoracic surgeon in the main or accident and emergency operating theatre. If the object is above the larynx and if an ENT surgeon or anaesthetist is not immediately available and the child is deteriorating the safest treatment is to insert a wide needle, such as Medicut size 14, into the trachea in the midline just below the thyroid cartilage. It may be preferable to insert two needles. No attempt should be made to look at the mouth or throat or remove the object, as the struggling that may follow may impact the object and prove fatal. The child should remain in the position he finds most comfortable, which is usually upright. Forceful attempts to make the child lie flat, for example for a radiograph, may result in complete airway obstruction.

BRONCHIAL ASTHMA

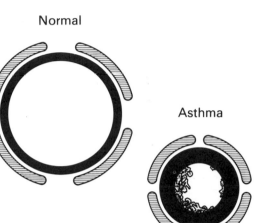

Normal

Asthma

The symptoms of bronchial asthma are caused by narrowing of the bronchi and bronchioles by mucosal swelling and contraction of the muscle in their walls, with viscid secretion obstructing the lumen. The muscle contraction is reversible by bronchodilators which belong to two main groups: β adrenoceptor stimulants such as salbutamol or xanthine derivatives such as aminophylline. In most children with bronchial asthma there are no symptoms or abnormal signs between acute attacks, and lung function tests, unless performed after exercise, are normal. Asthma is the most common chronic disease of childhood and it affects about 10% of schoolchildren. About 80% of children with asthma have the first symptoms before the age of 5 years and at least half will stop having attacks when they become adults.

During the past 20 years new prophylactic drugs and better methods of administering them have resulted in many children with asthma being completely free of symptoms. Treatment needs to be reviewed regularly as the severity fluctuates and the most suitable preparation changes as the child grows.

Diagnosis

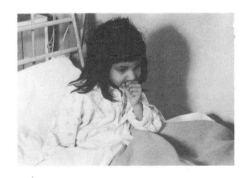

Bronchial asthma should be suspected if there is *recurrent* cough, wheezing, or shortness of breath, especially after exercise or during the night. Improvement with a bronchodilator is helpful evidence. The first attack may occur at any age, but to avoid many children with an acute lower respiratory tract infection being labelled as asthmatic it is preferable to wait until three episodes have occurred within a year before confirming the diagnosis. There is no clinical or laboratory method of distinguishing between acute bronchial infection and asthma. Rhonchi may be heard in the chest during and between attacks of asthma, but there may be no abnormal signs despite repeated examinations. Recurrent night cough may be the only feature, and the absence of night cough is the best evidence that treatment is adequate. The length of absences from school, poor growth, and chest deformity as well as the number of hospital admissions give an indication of the severity of the problem. Details of previous drug treatments may help to avoid the repetition of failures.

Assessment

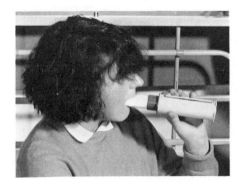

A detailed history should be taken of exposure to household pets or other animals which may belong to friends or relatives. Severe symptoms or hay fever at a particular time of the year may incriminate pollen. Skin tests tend to be negative under the age of 5 years and also when the child is taking steroids. The results may be helpful in avoiding exposure to allergens, but the long-term effects of attempts at desensitisation are unknown.

The single most useful test is the peak flow reading, which can be measured using the low-range (30–370 l/m) mini-Wright peak flow meter. Normal ranges are related to the height of the child. In asthma peak flow varies greatly throughout the day, being lowest in the early morning and shortly after five minutes of exercise. This exercise can be of any type. In childen over the age of 5 years, especially in those

Bronchial asthma

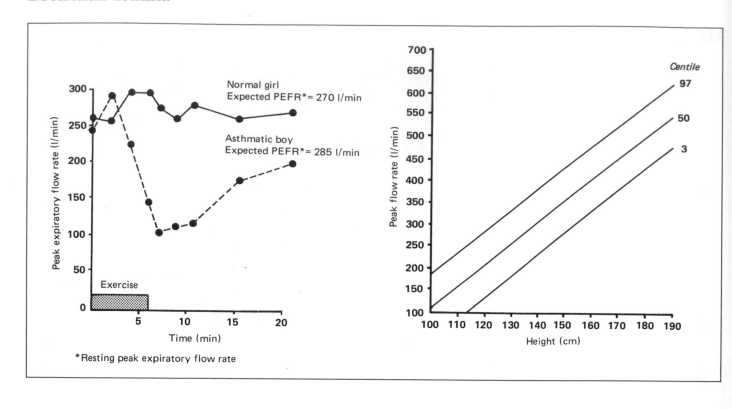

*Resting peak expiratory flow rate

in whom the diagnosis is not clear, a fall in peak expiratory flow rate of 15% or more after exercise or a similar rise with a bronchodilator confirms the diagnosis. About 10% of children with asthma have a normal response to these tests. Regular peak flow reading and completion of a standard diary card of symptoms may be helpful in assessing the severity of the problem and the response to treatment.

A chest radiograph is taken at the initial assessment to exclude a foreign body in the lung or oesophagus, but further films are usually not helpful. A sweat test excludes cystic fibrosis.

The importance of psychological factors in inducing attacks of asthma is difficult to determine, though stresses caused by absence from school, disruption of the family, and conflicting advice are inevitable in the severely affected child. The help given by a child psychiatrist may depend on his enthusiasm. The problem of the child who has had a recent increase in attacks or who is poorly controlled despite apparently adequate treatment should be discussed by the paediatrician with a child psychiatrist. Virus infections are the most important precipitating cause of attacks of asthma and antibiotics are therefore not indicated except for selected patients with severe attacks requiring hospital admission.

Date this card was started:		1	2	3	4	5	6	7	8	9	10
1. WHEEZE LAST NIGHT	Good night .... 0 Slept well but slightly wheezy .... 1 Woke x 2-3 because of wheeze .... 2 Bad night, awake most of time 3										
2. COUGH LAST NIGHT	None .... 0 Little .... 1 Moderately bad .... 2 Severe 3										
3. WHEEZE TODAY	None .... 0 Little .... 1 Moderately bad .... 2 Severe 3										
4. ACTIVITY TODAY	Quite normal .... 0 Can only run short distance .... 1 Limited to walking because of chest .... 2 Too breathless to walk 3										
5. NASAL SYMPTOMS	None .... 0 Mild .... 1 Moderate .... 2 Severe 3										
6. METER Best of 3 blows	Before breakfast Medicines .... Before bedtime Medicines										
7. DRUGS Number of doses actually taken during the past 24 hours.	Name of Drug / Dose Prescribed										
8. COMMENTS	Note if you see a Doctor (D) or stay away from school (S) or work (W) because of your chest and anything else important such as an infection (I).										

Allergen avoidance

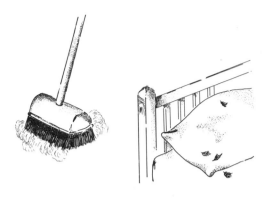

House dust, house dust mite, and grass pollens produce the highest incidence of positive skin tests in children with bronchial asthma. Complete avoidance of house dust is impossible but feather pillows can be replaced by foam rubber pillows and the mattress can be completely enclosed in a plastic bag. It may be helpful for a damp duster to be used for wiping surfaces and for cleaning in the child's room to take place while he is in another part of the house. Vinyl floor covering can be used instead of carpets. Fitted carpets are an important source of the house dust mite.

The importance of food in precipitating attacks and the value of exclusion diets in preventing symptoms are controversial. Recent studies suggest that the following items have precipitated symptoms in specific children: orange and lemon squash, fried foods, nuts, and drinks containing ice or carbon dioxide. If parents have noted that symptoms are precipitated by a particular food it would seem reasonable to avoid that food for a limited trial period of six weeks, but it is essential that this diet is supervised by a paediatric dietitian.

Drug treatment

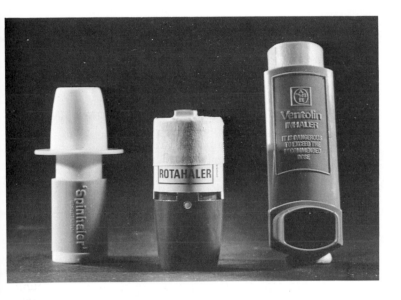

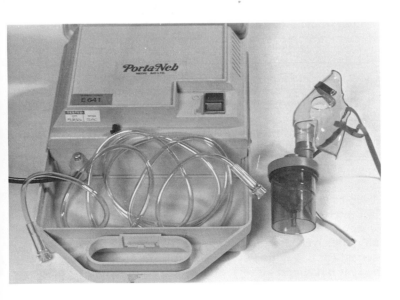

Selection of a route of administration which is appropriate to the age of the child is essential for effective treatment. A common cause of failure to respond to an inhaled drug is lack of proper tuition, and it is helpful if a practice nurse or health visitor takes on this task for all the children in the practice. Bronchodilator drugs can be given at any age, but they tend to be less effective in infants under the age of 18 months. Powder preparations can be inhaled by children over about 4 years of age. Pressurised canisters can be used by a child over about 10 years. It is essential that his coordination of inspiration and release of the dose is checked. The metered dose can be released into a plastic disposable cup or plastic container and younger children can inhale the drug through a valve, but this technique may not be effective.

Infrequent mild attacks (one in three months) can be treated by a bronchodilator given at the beginning of an upper respiratory tract infection and continued for a week. A β stimulant bronchodilator should also be given half an hour before vigorous exercise.

Children who have frequent attacks (more than once in six weeks) need a prophylactic drug continuously for at least a year. The choice is between sodium cromoglycate and long-acting theophylline preparations. Sodium cromoglycate has been used for over 15 years and the rare side effect is a cough during inhalation of the powder which can be eliminated by a preceding dose of bronchodilator. Children usually have to be over the age of 4 years before they can grasp the idea of sucking in air and powdered cromoglycate through the Spinhaler into their lungs. A whistle device can be attached to the Spinhaler to check correct technique. For younger children and those who cannot manage the powder, cromoglycate is available as a liquid preparation given as an aerosol. This needs a mains pump, which costs about £85, and the procedure takes about five minutes on each occasion. Hand operated nebulisers are not effective.

Bronchial asthma

Salbutamol

Cromoglycate ← → Theophylline

Steroid by inhalation

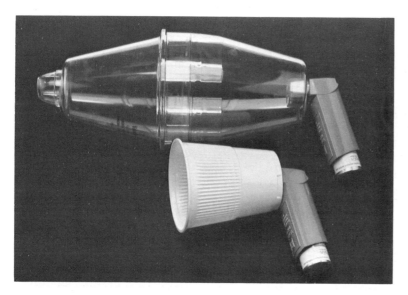

During the past eight years long-acting oral preparations of theophylline have been introduced into paediatric practice. Aminophylline contains theophylline and ethylenediamine. These preparations have a therapeutic effect for 10 hours or more, whereas the older preparations were effective for only about three hours owing to rapid elimination in children. Prescribing the exact dose is difficult as there is no liquid preparation; the tablets should not be broken and dividing a capsule does not provide an accurate dose. Neither the tablets nor the granules in the capsules should be chewed. The capsules can be opened and sprinkled on jam or given with milk. The doses in children are relatively high compared with those for adults, and blood concentrations must be measured to avoid the side effects of vomiting and headache.

Failure to respond to cromoglycate or theophylline is an indication for prophylactic inhaled steriods. As there have been no very long term studies of the effects of this treatment, there must be good indications before it is started. Beclomethasone dipropionate powder can be inhaled by children above the age of about 4 years using a Rotahaler. An alternative is budesonide, but this is available only as a pressured aerosol canister. The dose is released into a container and is inhaled by the child through a valve.

A few patients who are well controlled with prophylactic drugs need two or three courses of daily oral steriods each year. Each course should last less than a week and be confined to the known vulnerable seasons for that child. Oral steroids given on alternate mornings are still needed for a few children who have failed to respond to all other forms of treatment.

Children taking prophylactic drugs should always have available a fast-acting bronchodilator to treat acute attacks.

Acute attack of asthma

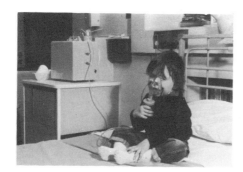

If an acute asthma attack does not respond quickly to the child's usual treatment at home he will need urgent treatment with salbutamol or terbutaline aerosol using a face mask and nebuliser attached to an air compressor or compressed oxygen supply. If the family doctor is not immediately available to provide this treatment the child should be seen in the day care unit or accident and emergency department. Delay in appreciating the severity of the attack or providing treatment can be fatal. Drowsiness, cyanosis of the lips, and shortness of breath during speaking are signs of a severe attack. The duration of the episode of asthma and details of the drugs taken previously should be noted, especially those taken during the preceding 24 hours. Tachycardia is often a side effect of drugs.

Nebulised bronchodilator drugs can be given to children of any age and are accepted if the mask is held by the mother and she talks to the child during treatment. The mother's presence calms the child. He has usually improved considerably before the dose is finished. He is then observed for 2–4 hours. If he is completely well after that time he can be sent home and be reviewed by the family doctor or paediatrician. In children old enough to use a peak flow meter the response to treatment can be monitored and failure to improve after the bronchodilator or a peak flow rate of less than 25% of that expected is an indication for admission.

Treatment on admission

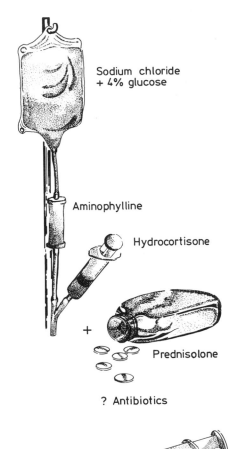

Sodium chloride + 4% glucose

Aminophylline

Hydrocortisone

+

Prednisolone

? Antibiotics

PO₂   PCO₂

On the way he should be encouraged to sit upright in the position that makes him most comfortable; this is usually with his elbows forward. If two hours have elapsed since the previous dose of nebulised salbutamol a further dose may be given with oxygen. Alternatively, nebulised ipratropium bromide can be given. These drugs can have an additive therapeutic effect and may be given alternately or together. If he is deteriorating the following are given.

(1) Intravenous fluids are started with sodium chloride 0·18% with glucose 4%. In addition to the maintenance volume extra fluid may be needed as the child may be dehydrated.

(2) If an aminophylline preparation has not been given during the previous 24 hours a single intravenous dose of 3 to 5 mg/kg body weight can be given. It must be given slowly by adding it to the burette of the giving set and allowing it to run in over at least half an hour. This is followed by an infusion of aminophylline at a lower dose of 1 mg/kg/hour for a further eight hours. If aminophylline has been given during the previous 24 hours the initial large dose is omitted and the slow infusion given.

(3) Hydrocortisone is given in a dose of 100 mg intravenously every three hours for three doses and then every six hours for a total of 24 hours. The dose is not related to body weight.

(4) Prednisolone 2 mg/kg/24 hours by mouth should replace the intravenous hydrocortisone as soon as the child can swallow. This is gradually reduced and stopped within a week.

(5) Humidified oxygen at a concentration of 100% is given by face mask or other method acceptable to the child.

(6) If the child is drowsy or becoming exhausted he should be admitted to the intensive care unit, where arterial blood needs to be taken for urgent estimation of PaO_2, $PaCO_2$, pH, and plasma sodium and potassium concentrations. The most suitable site for obtaining arterial blood is the radial artery, and the femoral artery should be avoided. Deterioration may occur rapidly and the same observer should see the patient at least every half hour. These investigations need to be repeated every two hours or whenever the child's condition becomes worse. Artificial ventilation is indicated if the $PaCO_2$ is rising rapidly or is above 9 kPa (67 mm Hg). Steroids do not have a maximal effect before six to eight hours.

If the attack is severe and does not respond quickly to treatment a chest radiograph should be performed to exclude pneumothorax or pneumonia.

Suggested drug doses

Adrenoceptor stimulants

(1) Salbutamol (Ventolin)
Oral	1–2 years	1 mg per dose × 3 daily
	2–8 years	1–2 mg per dose × 3 daily
	over 8 years	4 mg per dose × 3 daily
Powder (rotacaps)		200 µg × 3 daily

Nebulised (with pump) 2.5–5.0 mg to be repeated *once* only after 4 hours (if the child is being treated at home)

(2) Terbutaline (Bricanyl)
Oral	1–2 years	0.75 mg per dose × 3 daily
	2–8 years	1.5–2.5 mg per dose × 3 daily
	over 8 years	2.5–5.0 mg per dose × 3 daily

Nebulised (with pump) 2 mg to be repeated *once* only after 4 hours (if the child is being treated at home)

Xanthine derivatives

(3) Aminophylline tablets (Phyllocontin)   8–10 mg/kg dose

(4) Theophylline capsules (Slo-phyllin)   12 hourly

Cromoglycate

(5) Sodium cromoglycate (Intal)
Powder	1 capsule (20 mg) × 3 daily
Nebulised (with pump)	1 ampoule (20 mg) × 3 daily

Steroid

(6) Beclomethasone dipropionate (Becotide)
Powder	5–10 years	100 µg × 3 daily
	over 10 years	200 µg × 3 daily

ACUTE ABDOMINAL PAIN

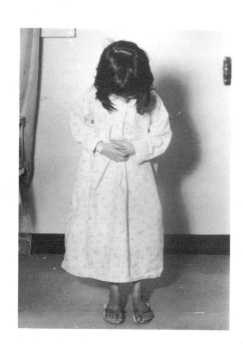

Causes
Surgical
Medical
Gastroenteritis
?

At the beginning of an episode of abdominal pain it may be difficult to make an exact diagnosis. The picture will become clearer if the child is seen again after a few hours, but if this is not possible the child may have to be admitted to hospital for observation. Many parents are worried that their child has acute appendicitis, and the responsibility for keeping an eye on the child should not be left to the parents, who do not have the knowledge to make the right judgments.

Although a definite diagnosis should be attempted it is essential to place the patient in one of the following groups:
(a) surgical problem: admit;
(b) chronic medical problem: admit or arrange paediatric appointment;
(c) gastroenteritis: manage at home or admit to an isolation cubicle of the paediatric unit depending on the severity of the illness;
(d) acute non-specific abdominal pain;
(e) cause uncertain: see again within a few hours or admit to hospital for observation.

Appendicitis may produce features suggestive of many other conditions and it may not be possible to make a firm diagnosis or to exclude it on one observation. If surgical intervention is a possibility the parents should be warned not to give their child any food or drink in the meantime.

Although the mother gives the details of the history, it is important to obtain as much information as possible from the child himself. Children under the age of 3 years may, however, point to the abdomen as the site of pain when in fact the cause of the symptoms is in another area such as the throat. Abdominal tenderness can be observed even in small children, who may push away the examiner's hands.

The site and duration of the pain should be noted and whether previous attacks have occurred. The duration and severity of diarrhoea or vomiting should be noted. There may be fever, rash, or pain in the joints.

Appendicitis

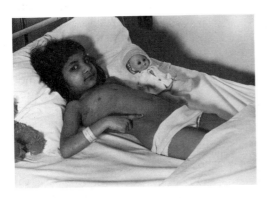

The wall of the appendix is thinner in a child than in an adult; the omentum is less developed and perforation is often followed by generalised peritonitis. The child himself should be asked about his pain. Older children can often localise their pain accurately if they are asked to point to the pain with one finger. Pain around the umbilicus often starts suddenly and is followed by vomiting. The pain may be intermittent or continuous and colicky or dull. It may be relieved during sleep. After a few hours, during which there may be some improvement, the pain moves to the right iliac fossa. In about a quarter of patients the pain is in the right iliac fossa from the beginning. A child with appendicitis may have constipation or diarrhoea. His temperature may be raised. The child usually lies still as his pain is aggravated by movement. Movements of the abdominal wall during breathing are restricted.

Appendicitis is extremely difficult to diagnose in infants less than 2 years of age and perforation often occurs before the diagnosis is made. Then the infant looks extremely ill and has considerable abdominal tenderness.

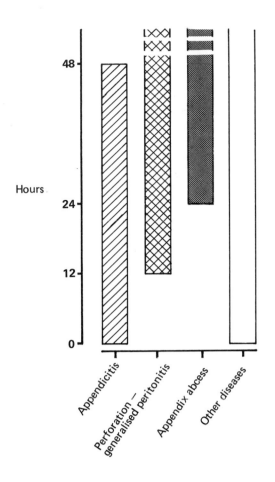

Hours

The bladder should be emptied before the abdomen is examined. The abdomen should be palpated gently with a warm hand or the bell end of a stethoscope, beginning in the *left* iliac fossa. Tenderness is detected by change of expression on the child's face, and is localised to the right iliac fossa before perforation. Guarding is significant only if the child is completely relaxed. Bowel sounds are reduced if perforation has already occurred. Rectal examination should be performed only once and it is better to leave it to the surgeon. Very gentle examination is necessary to determine local tenderness rectally. The fact that a rectal examination has not been performed should be recorded in the patient's notes.

If the appendix is situated in the pelvis or behind the caecum diagnosis is particularly difficult. Tenderness may be shown only on deep palpation and there may be diarrhoea or urinary symptoms, but there is no excess of pus cells in the urine microscopically.

A full physical examination should be done to exclude disease in another organ, especially the respiratory system, as it may be responsible for the symptoms. The white cell count is not helpful and need not be considered as a routine test for children with suspected appendicitis. Microscopy of the urine should be carried out immediately if there is any doubt about the diagnosis and chest radiography should be considered.

If a definite diagnosis cannot be made initially the child should be examined several times during the first 24 hours of his pain because perforation is more likely if the pain has been present longer than that period. If the pain pasts longer than 48 hours the child is likely to have generalised peritonitis, an appendix abscess, or pain not related to the appendix. If an episode of pain lasts continuously for longer than six hours the patient should be examined again.

Acute appendicitis and the other diagnoses discussed below should be considered in every child with acute abdominal pain. But in most children the cause cannot be found. The final diagnosis has been termed "acute non-specific abdominal pain" and suggestive features include intermittent central abdominal pain and tenderness without guarding lasting 24–36 hours. Sore throat, pyrexia, or vomiting may be present. Clusters of cases suggest that there are infectious causes.

Intussusception

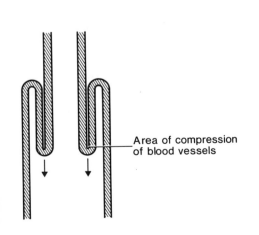

Area of compression of blood vessels

An intussusception is a partial or complete intestinal obstruction due to invagination of a proximal portion of the gut into a more distal portion. It may occur at any age although the maximum incidence is at 3–11 months. An intussusception may be easily diagnosed in a child who has all the typical features but these children are not common. The distinctive feature is the periodicity of the attacks, which may consist of severe screaming, drawing up of the legs, and severe pallor. Some episodes consist of pallor alone. The attack lasts a few minutes and then disappears, to recur about 20 minutes later, though attacks may be more frequent. One or two loose stools may be passed initially, suggesting a diagnosis of acute gastroenteritis. Blood-stained mucus may be passed rectally or shown by rectal examination. But some patients pass no blood rectally. Between attacks the infant appears normal and there may be no abnormal signs apart from a palpable mass.

It is difficult to examine the abdomen during an attack because the child cries continuously, but between attacks a mass, most commonly in the right upper quadrant, can be felt in 70% of children. If the diagnosis is definite some surgeons prefer to carry out a laparotomy without further investigations. If the history is short others arrange an urgent barium enema examination, which may reduce the intussusception. A barium enema is helpful when the diagnosis is uncertain but it should not be performed if there is clinical or radiological evidence of complete intestinal obstruction because there is a risk of perforating the intestine. In about 6% of cases there is a persisting mechanical cause of the intussusception and this will not be detected by the barium enema.

Inguinal hernia and torsion of testis

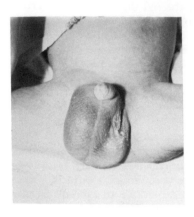

Strangulation of an inguinal hernia is likely to be present if the hernia is not reducible easily and there is abdominal pain. Gangrene of an area of small intestine may already have occurred and this part may have to be resected. The danger of strangulation of an inguinal hernia in infants under 2 years is considerably greater than at any other time, and any infant with an inguinal hernia must therefore be admitted for early operation. There is no place for conservative treatment.

The genitalia should be examined in every child with abdominal pain: 25% of cases of testicular torsion present initially with lower abdominal, rather than testicular, pain. A swollen tender testis should be assumed to be a torsion of the testis as orchitis is rare unless the child has mumps. An urgent surgical opinion should be obtained.

Other causes

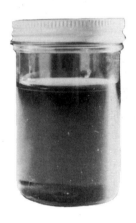

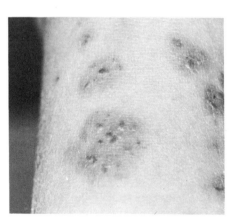

Urinary tract infection—In children with urinary tract infections the pain is usually in one loin but may be central. There may be fever, but dysuria and frequency of micturition are uncommon in younger children. Rarely haematuria may be present. Microscopy of the urine should be carried out immediately and the child admitted for confirmation of the diagnosis if organisms or an excessive number of pus cells are present in the urine.

Trauma—If the patient has been in a car crash or had an injury to the abdomen within the previous week the possibility of a ruptured viscus such as the spleen should be considered.

Henoch-Schönlein purpura—Abdominal pain may precede but usually accompanies the rash and joint swelling of Henoch–Schönlein purpura. The rash, which consists of haemorrhagic papules as well as purpuric spots, appears on the extensor surfaces of the limbs and the buttocks but spares the trunk. Blood may be passed rectally.

Diabetic ketoacidosis—Children with ketoacidosis may have abdominal pain which resolves during treatment with insulin and intravenous fluids. The diagnosis can be excluded by finding a normal blood glucose concentration with a BM stix test or by finding no glucose in the urine.

Sickle-cell disease—Painful "crises" occur as a result of occlusion of small blood vessels with distal ischaemia and infarction. Abdominal pain may be due to occlusion of intestinal or splenic vessels. Other organs commonly affected are the small bones of the hands and feet and the pulmonary vessels. Any child of African or Mediterranean origin who has obscure abdominal pain should have a sickle-cell test performed as an emergency and be admitted to hospital.

Recurrent abdominal pain of childhood—At least 10% of schoolchildren suffer recurrent abdominal pain—or the periodic syndrome. The condition should be diagnosed only in children who have had at least three episodes of pain over longer than three months. Two-thirds of the patients have a history of vomiting associated with abdominal pain. There is no abdominal tenderness. The child with recurrent abdominal pain of childhood is just as susceptible as any other child to physical disease, such as appendicitis. If the pain is present continuously for longer than six hours an organic cause must be considered (see next chapter for further details of recurrent abdominal pain of childhood).

Gastroenteritis—Gastroenteritis sometimes presents with abdominal pain as the main symptom and it will be discussed in the chapter on vomiting and diarrhoea.

Sickle cell

RECURRENT ABDOMINAL PAIN

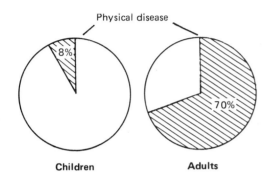

Physical disease

8%

70%

Children   Adults

Recurrent abdominal pain, which is also called the periodic syndrome or abdominal migraine, is diagnosed on the basis of at least three episodes of pain in over three months. At least 10% of schoolchildren have recurrent abdominal pain. The symptoms usually begin at the age of 5 years, though they may appear as early as 2 years or as late as 13 years. In a study of 100 children investigated in hospital only eight were found to have organic causes for the pain, including three with renal problems. In contrast, 70% of adults with recurrent abdominal pain have a demonstrable physical cause: most have a peptic ulcer, which is uncommon in children, or disease of the biliary tract, which is extremely rare in childhood.

In children with recurrent abdominal pain the commonest emotional state is anxiety and the commonest trigger for attacks of pain is events at school.

History

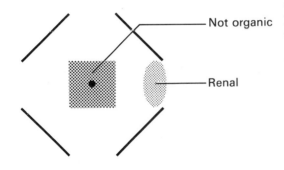

— Not organic

— Renal

Details of the first attack may be remembered with special clarity and may help to elucidate the cause. Two-thirds of the children have central abdominal pain, which is usually not organic in origin, but pain in other sites may have a physical cause. Pain on one side of the abdomen suggests renal disease. Aggravating and relieving factors should be considered but the type of pain is usually not helpful, and very severe pain causing the child to cry out may still derive from emotional causes. The duration and frequency of the pain and whether it occurs on a particular day of the week, at weekends, or holidays are all important.

About two-thirds of the children have vomiting with the pain and 10% have diarrhoea during attacks. Twenty-five per cent have headaches and 10% pain in their limbs between attacks. Pallor during an attack is noticed in half the cases, and a quarter of children are sleepy after an attack.

Emotional and social factors

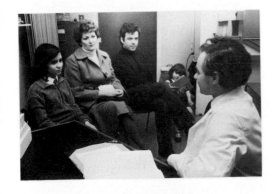

In the parents and siblings of the children with recurrent abdominal pain the incidence of similar complaints is nearly six times higher than in those of controls. The family member most often affected is the mother. There may be a history of domestic difficulties or parental illness, including depression. Parents should be asked what sort of child their son or daughter is and what disorder they particularly fear in their child. Their reactions to the child should be observed during the visit. The child's attitude to the rest of his family and his friends may need to be explored. The parents must be encouraged to say what they feel, and apparently irrelevant details about everyday life at home and at school may be of diagnostic importance.

Recurrent abdominal pain

Physical disease

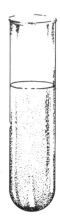

Microscopy

Culture

Diastix

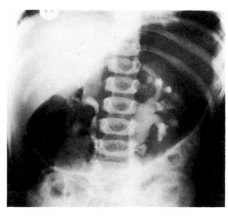

Parents as well as doctors are worried about missing physical disease in children with recurrent abdominal pain. A thorough initial clinical examination reassures the parents and should be repeated during an attack if an opportunity arises. For most children all the investigations can be arranged at the first visit so that long-term management can be planned at the second interview.

A specimen of urine should be sent to the laboratory for examination by microscopy and culture from *every* child with recurrent abdominal pain. If the pain is central and there are no abnormal signs no further investigations are needed. Pain in the lateral part of the abdomen should be investigated by ultrasound examination of the kidneys, bladder, pancreas, and gallbladder. Plain radiographs of the abdomen will show the majority of renal stones or calcification in the pancreas. The management of upper abdominal pain is controversial but if it does not improve after two months of observation it may be necessary to exclude a peptic ulcer by barium meal examination and gastroscopy and chronic pancreatitis by a radiograph of the abdomen for calcification.

Recurrent abdominal pain and pronounced weight loss suggest the possibility of Crohn's disease but confirmation may require barium studies, sigmoidoscopy and possibly colonoscopy.

Abdominal distension during episodes of pain may be due to volvulus with associated malrotation of the gut, and a plain radiograph of the abdomen with the patient erect during an attack is needed. A barium study may help to confirm the diagnosis. If pain is localised to the right hypochondrium investigations for gall bladder disease should be considered.

Recurrent episodes of acute appendicitis are a rare cause of recurrent abdominal pain.

Discussions with child and parents

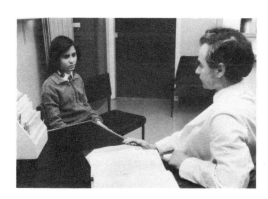

Ideally the child should be seen by himself as well as with both parents at the first visit to explore his feelings about his abdominal pain. At the end of the first interview the most likely diagnosis is discussed with the whole group. If the pain seems to have an emotional origin it is best to explain that a large proportion of children as well as some adults have abdominal pain which has no organic cause but which is precipitated by emotional factors. It is important to mention that the child does experience pain, which may be severe, and that he is not pretending. It is helpful to explain that the physical and emotional causes are being explored together and that the child will be reviewed regularly until the pain disappears or has considerably improved. The parents should be asked for their permission for a school report to be requested.

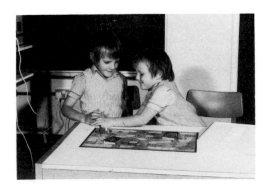

At the second visit it is essential to convince the parents that the likely causes of organic disease have been excluded. The parents may have recollected important details as a result of promptings at the previous visit, or the teacher or family may have discovered a remediable factor at school. The child may be bullied at school, or chance remarks which appear innocuous to a teacher may have a devastating effect on a child. Alternatively a child may feel very hurt by not being given praise when he thinks it is due. Children are very sensitive to injustice and may treat their teachers as gods. The excessive ambition of parents, excessive homework, or going to a large middle school after a small village school may all produce severe stress. Parental discord or separation may be bewildering to a small child. The child who behaves superbly in class may show his mother the results of his pent-up tension.

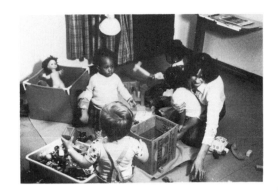

By guidance the parents can be shown how to modify the child's environment to help his adaptation. Practical and tactful advice is needed for the inadequate mother who makes excessive emotional demands on her child or for a father who loads the child with his own ambitions. In advising them it is helpful to try to discover why they feel that way. The child cannot be insulated from all stresses but sources of excessive tension should be removed.

Children who have pain every day may need to be admitted to hospital for a short period to take the stress off the family. The object is to determine whether changes in environment will affect the pain, and the opportunity should not be used to carry out an excessive number of investigations. The pain usually abates in hospital, though not always, but may become worse again immediately after the child returns home.

Children with recurrent abdominal pain of emotional origin may also develop physical disease such as acute appendicitis, and if the pain lasts continuously for more than six hours the child should be seen again by a doctor as an emergency.

Prognosis

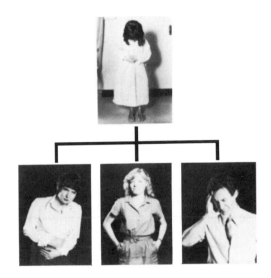

A high proportion of adolescents and young adults who have attended hospital with recurrent abdominal pain in childhood are later found to have continuing symptoms. In one study about a third were found to have continuing attacks of abdominal pain. One-third were completely free of symptoms, while in a third abdominal pain had ceased but other symptoms such as recurrent headache had developed. Recurrent abdominal pain in childhood may not be as benign as previously believed but may delineate a group of children who find it difficult to adapt to their environment both as children and as adults.

VOMITING AND ACUTE DIARRHOEA

Causes of vomiting
1 Acute gastroenteritis
2 Acute otitis media
3 Periodic syndrome
4 Urinary tract infection
5 Onset of acute appendicitis or intussusception
6 Intestinal obstruction
7 Whooping cough
8 Meningitis
9 Infectious hepatitis

Doctors should always be worried about vomiting in a young child. Although it may herald only the onset of a less serious illness, such as acute otitis media, vomiting may be the first symptom of a potentially lethal disease such as meningitis or intestinal obstruction. The child needs to be seen urgently if the vomitus is bile-stained (suggesting intestinal obstruction) or if he is drowsy or refusing feeds, which may occur in meningitis. Diagnosis over the telephone without seeing a vomiting child may be disastrous. By the age of 1 year regurgitation of feeds has usually stopped, and vomiting signifies a new illness.

Whooping cough

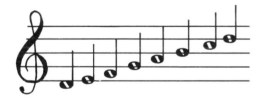

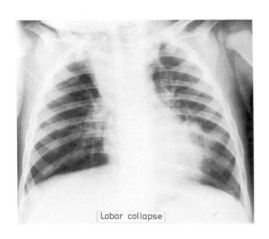

Lobar collapse

Vomiting may be so severe in infants with whooping cough that the mother is more worried by the vomiting than the cough. During the first one or two weeks of the illness (catarrhal phase) there is a short dry nocturnal cough. Later, bouts of 10 to 20 short coughs occur both day and night. The cough is dry and each cough is on the same high note or goes up in a musical scale. Vomiting may occur towards the end of a long attack of coughing. The coughing is followed by a sharp indrawing of breath, which causes the whoop. Some children with proved pertussis infection never develop the whoop. Feeding often provokes a spasm of coughing, which may culminate in vomiting. Afterwards there is a short period when the child can be fed again without provoking more coughing. In uncomplicated cases there are no abnormal signs in the respiratory system.

Whooping cough may occur in children who have been fully immunised against it. *Bordetella pertussis* may be isolated from a pernasal swab, which should be plated on a special culture medium immediately after being taken. A blood lymphocyte count of over $10 \times 10^9/1$ with a normal erythrocyte sedimentation rate suggests whooping cough. A seven-day course of oral erythromycin, ampicillin, or amoxycillin reduces the infectivity of the patient but does not usually affect the course of the disease if vomiting has already started. Symptomatic treatment with promethazine, salbutamol, or phenobarbitone to try to reduce the cough usually has little effect, and the parents can be consoled only by being told that the vomiting will eventually stop.

If there are abnormal signs in the respiratory system, the child becomes generally ill, or the cough persists longer than six weeks a chest radiograph is necessary to exclude the secondary complications of bronchopneumonia or lobar collapse, which need treatment with physiotherapy and antibiotics. If the coughing attacks are severe admission to hospital may be necessary. Ideally a child should be admitted with his mother to an isolation room on the children's ward.

Meningitis

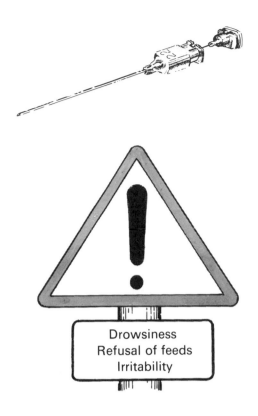

Drowsiness
Refusal of feeds
Irritability

In children aged under 3 years it is difficult to recognise early signs of meningitis. There may be fever, vomiting, irritability, a high-pitched cry, and convulsions. Refusal of feeds and drowsiness are ominous signs. Neck stiffness may be difficult to detect.

Older children may have fever, vomiting, and severe headache, but irritability, drowsiness, and unusual behaviour are more useful features. To detect neck stiffness the degree of flexion of the neck is observed when the child is asked to look at his umbilicus. If there is any doubt an attempt can be made to flex the head gently. A test for older children is Kernig's sign, which is present if there is pronounced resistance to extension of the knee when the patient is supine with both the thigh and knee flexed.

A purpuric rash suggests meningococcal infection, and an immediate intravenous or intramuscular injection of 300 mg of benzylpenicillin is needed.

The highest incidence of meningitis occurs between 6 and 12 months of age and the younger the child the more difficult the diagnosis. A useful rule is that if a doctor thinks that a lumbar puncture might be needed, it should be done. If papilloedema is present the child should be transferred to a neurosurgical unit before lumbar puncture is attempted. Except in patients with a purpuric rash no antibiotics should be given before the lumbar puncture is performed. Every child with meningitis needs intravenous fluids and antibiotics given by bolus injection into the infusion line. Chloramphenicol should be used when the meningitis is due to *Haemophilus influenzae* or when no organism can be identified on the smear of cerebrospinal fluid. High doses of intravenous penicillin G are used for meningococcal, pneumococcal, or streptococcal infection. Intrathecal penicillin has no place in treatment and may be lethal.

Acute gastroenteritis

Dehydration

Electrolyte abnormalities

Cross infection

Diarrhoea is the passage of loose stools more often than usual. When diarrhoea is severe the stools may be mistaken for urine. When this is a possibility a urine bag should be placed in position and the child nursed on a sheet of polyethylene. Acute gastroenteritis is the most common cause of acute diarrhoea.

Acute gastroenteritis is an acute infection mainly affecting the small intestine which causes diarrhoea with or without vomiting. In children aged over 3 years abdominal pain may be a prominent feature. The main danger is dehydration and electrolyte imbalance, but the infant may also be very infectious for other infants in a ward or nursery. Gastroenteritis is particularly dangerous to infants aged under 2 years.

Early signs of dehydration are often difficult to detect, particularly in fat toddlers, but recent weight loss is often a valuable indicator. Sunken eyes, inelastic skin, and a dry tongue are late signs, but if the infant has not passed urine for several hours severe dehydration is probable. The infant must be examined in detail to exclude any other acute infections.

The rotavirus is the commonest cause of gastroenteritis in infants and children throughout the world. It affects every age group and easily spreads throughout a family, although adults usually have no symptoms but are often carriers of rotavirus. Several distinct episodes of diarrhoea can be due to the rotavirus as there are several serotypes. The incubation period is 24 to 48 hours and a respiratory illness, including acute otitis media, precedes the gastrointestinal symptoms in about half the patients. Vomiting which lasts for one to three days is followed by abnormal stools for about five days. Treatment is aimed at keeping the child well hydrated until he recovers spontaneously. The frequency of the stools falls with effective treatment but the consistency of the stools remains abnormal for about a week.

If the patient is given an antibiotic early in the illness subsequent diarrhoea may be attributed to the antibiotic rather than to the rotavirus infection.

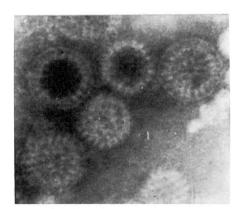

Vomiting and acute diarrhoea

Management

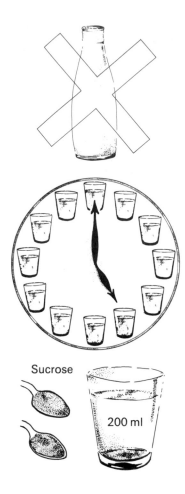

Sucrose

200 ml

Clinical signs of severe dehydration or the loss of 5% or more of body weight are definite indications for admission. If the infant relapses after treatment or social problems prevent him being treated at home he should also be admitted. Infants who vomit persistently usually need to be admitted, though mild symptoms may be managed at home by giving frequent small volumes of liquid by mouth.

In mild cases the main principle of management is to stop milk and solids and give a glucose or sucrose solution orally. After 24 hours fruit or vegetable purées may be introduced and then other items from the child's normal diet. The mother should be asked not to give the child milk or milk products for three days and then to introduce them gradually. Vomiting may be reduced by giving small volumes of fluid every half hour or hour. The child should be allowed to drink as much as he wants but he needs at least 1 litre each 24 hours.

Kaolin should not be prescribed as it deflects the mother's attention from the main treatment. No antibiotics should be given to children with gastroenteritis treated at home.

In severe cases of dehydration or persistent vomiting oral fluids must be replaced with intravenous fluids in infants admitted to hospital. During the next day a third of the fluid requirement should be given as an oral glucose–electrolyte mixture, and later fruit and vegetable purées are introduced. Most children are discharged from hospital on normal diets within a week. Infants in hospital with diarrhoea must be barrier nursed in a cubicle, which should ideally be in an annexe to the children's ward.

The ideal oral rehydrating fluid is a glucose–electrolyte mixture, but a 5% glucose or 4% sucrose solution is easily available and safe. Single-dose sachets of glucose–electrolyte powder (Dioralyte) or glucose–sucrose–electrolyte powder (Rehydrat) are available, which enable mothers to make up the mixture accurately at home. A safe alternative is 4% sucrose solution, which can be made up by the mother using 2 level teaspoonfuls of granulated sucrose in 200 ml (6 oz) water. *It is dangerous for mothers to add salt to this mixture.*

Investigations

Microscopy
Stool culture
Rotavirus
Electron microscopy of stool
Plasma, sodium, potassium, and urea estimations

Ideally a stool should be sent to the laboratory for detection of pathogens, but this is not necessary for mild cases treated at home. Only a small proportion of children have bacteria such as pathogenic *Escherichia coli*, *Shigella*, *Salmonella*, or *Campylobacter* isolated from their stools. Recently cryptosporidium, which can be seen by light microscopy, has been shown to be a common pathogen. Most cases of gastroenteritis in children are caused by viruses, usually rotaviruses, and these can be identified by direct electron microscopy of the stool. Rotavirus can also be detected by a quick slide test which does not need electron microscopy.

Children needing intravenous fluids should have their plasma electrolyte, bicarbonate, and urea concentrations measured urgently.

If two or more infants in a ward or nursery have diarrhoea at the same time cross-infection should be presumed, even if their stool cultures show no pathogens. Stools from all the infants on the ward should be sent for culture and electron microscopy. Admissions to the ward may have to be stopped.

Progress

Date	Weight	Treatment
2·1·80	5·1 kg	Glucose–electrolyte mixture
2·1·80	5·4 kg	Glucose–electrolyte mixture
3·1·80	5·4 kg	

The infant must be seen again by the doctor within 12 hours of starting treatment to ensure that the illness is improving, the infant is not losing too much weight, and the mother understands the management. Severe dehydration can occur within a few hours, and it is helpful to have a specific policy to ensure adequate follow-up visits.

The main cause of relapse or persistent symptoms which demand admission to hospital is failure to follow a plan of treatment. A few infants aged under 2 years have temporary mucosal damage. This causes the diarrhoea to persist for longer than two weeks and is considered in the later chapter on chronic diarrhoea.

Gastroenteritis in developing countries

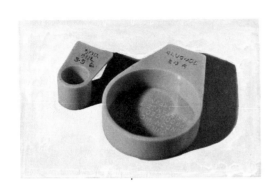

In developing countries the continuation of breast-feeding may be essential for survival. Although infants who are completely breast-fed rarely have severe gastroenteritis, weaning foods made up with water may infect a breast-fed infant. These infants can be managed by continuing the breast-feeding and supplementing the fluid intake to prevent dehydration until the infant spontaneously recovers. Supplements may be given by mouth in mild cases and intravenously in severe cases. An easier method is to give them by continuous intragastric infusion, for which the fluid does not have to be sterile.

Oral rehydrating fluids can be made up using specially designed spoons to measure the sugar and salt. Mothers and older siblings can be taught to use this mixture at the beginning of an episode of diarrhoea rather than wait until the child is dehydrated. Simple slogans such as "a cup of fluid for every stool" are effective.

CHRONIC DIARRHOEA

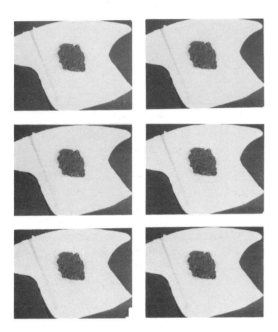

Diarrhoea which lasts longer than two weeks can be called chronic. To provide perspective, diarrhoea starting at any age will be discussed here. In Britain chronic diarrhoea with normal growth between the ages of 1 and 3 years is usually of no sinister significance. It is popularly known as "toddler diarrhoea" and is probably due to failure to chew food. In developing countries chronic diarrhoea is often caused by acute or chronic intestinal infection. In all parts of the world acute gastroenteritis may be followed by chronic diarrhoea, and the importance of cows' milk protein intolerance and secondary lactase deficiency as causes of this syndrome is controversial. Malabsorption may be presumed if there is chronic diarrhoea and the growth chart shows inadequate weight gain. Coeliac disease and cystic fibrosis are both uncommon; each occurs in about one in 2000 children. Crohn's disease is rare below the age of 7 years.

History and examination

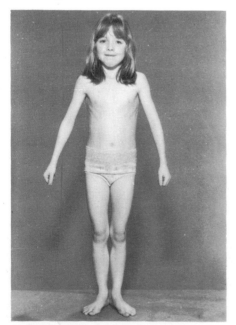

The history should include an inquiry about the duration of the symptoms; the frequency, consistency, and colour of the stools; and whether any fluid is present with the stools. The date when the first gluten was eaten and the detailed diet of an average day need to be recorded. The presence of recognisable foods such as beans, peas, or carrots in the stool is noted. Details of medicines and diets prescribed should be considered.

There are usually few abnormal signs. Abdominal distension and wasting, particularly of the inner aspects of the thighs and of the buttocks, should be noted.

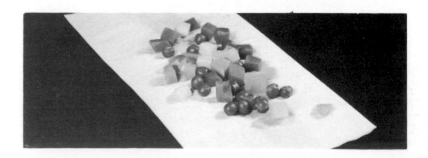

Investigations in children over 1 year with normal growth

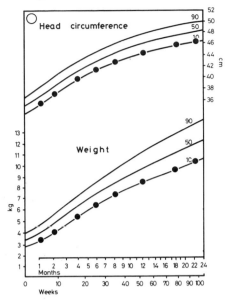

Growth as shown on a growth chart is the most valuable single investigation. The chart can often be completed from measurements already taken at the local clinic. If growth is normal severe malabsorption due to coeliac disease or cystic fibrosis is unlikely. A normal growth chart and the presence of recognisable food in the stools suggests that the child has toddler diarrhoea. This is probably due to failure to chew well and resolves spontaneously. Apart from examining the stools for pathogens, including *Giardia*, repeat measurements of growth are the only investigation required.

If no recognisable food is present in the stools cows' milk protein intolerance should be considered (see below).

Investigations in children under 1 year or those with poor weight gain

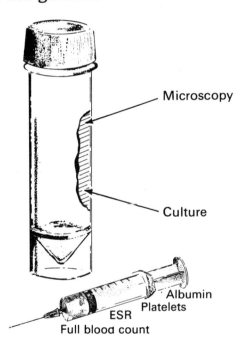

Microscopy

Culture

Albumin
Platelets
ESR
Full blood count

Sucrose   Lactose

The stool should be examined for parasites including *Giardia* and cryptosporidium and cultured for pathogens including pathogenic *Escherichia coli*. Blood is taken for a full blood count, erythrocyte sedimentation rate, platelet count, and plasma albumin estimation. A sweat test is performed and, if the result is normal, separate sucrose and lactose tolerance tests. (In some patients jejunal biopsy may be performed before sugar tolerance tests.) Severe diarrhoea during the 24 hours after a test dose of the sugar suggests intolerance, and the fluid part of the stool should be examined by Clinitest and sugar chromatography. A concentration of more than 0.5% of reducing substances in the stool indicates intolerance to that sugar. Serial blood glucose estimations during the tolerance tests are not performed because they give misleading results. All these tests can be carried out in the day care unit or outpatient department.

If the sweat test and tolerance tests are normal jejunal biopsy is considered. Some units carry out biopsies safely in the day care unit but others admit the child. Stool collections for fat excretion are no longer used as a screening test for coeliac disease. It is difficult to obtain complete collections of stool, and a poor appetite due to an infection caught in the ward often results in an inadequate fat intake. Most laboratories resent doing faecal fat estimations.

A completely flat mucosa on biopsy, devoid of villi, suggests that the child has coeliac disease. Similar abnormalities may be found in a wide variety of problems, including gastroenteritis, iron deficiency anaemia, malnutrition, and cows' milk protein intolerance. In these conditions the lesion may be patchy so that a single biopsy may fail to show an abnormal area.

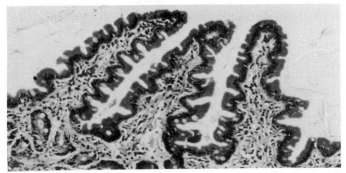
Normal

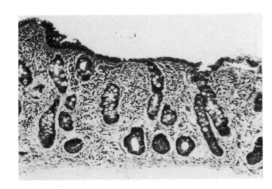

Chronic diarrhoea

Cows' milk protein intolerance

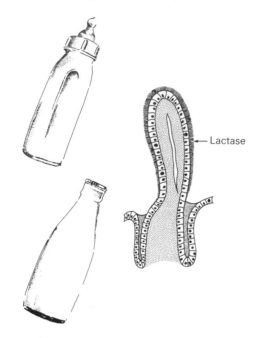

Lactase

The prevalence of intolerance to cows' milk protein varies widely according to different workers but is probably about one in 1000 infants. Diarrhoea starts between birth and 24 months. The intolerance resolves by the age of 2 years. Although many abnormalities have been described in laboratory tests none of the tests are easily available or reliable for routine clinical care. The diagnosis depends on withdrawing all products containing cows' milk and challenging the infant with 5 ml of milk while he is under supervision in a day care unit or ward. If severe diarrhoea occurs within 48 hours the diagnosis is confirmed and a cows' milk-free diet supervised by a dietitian prescribed. Infants under the age of 1 year may need a milk substitute and a soy-based preparation is often used, although up to half of these children eventually become intolerant of it. The cows' milk challenge is repeated every two to three months until the infant can tolerate it. The volume of milk given is doubled each day until normal amounts are received.

Infants with cows' milk protein intolerance may also have secondary lactase deficiency. This must be distinguished from isolated lactase deficiency of genetic origin, which causes diarrhoea after the age of 2 to 3 years. This type is extremely common in a variety of ethnic groups throughout the world but is not found in Caucasian races.

Cystic fibrosis

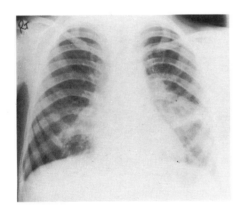

■● Cystic fibrosis
▨◉ Carrier
□○ Normal

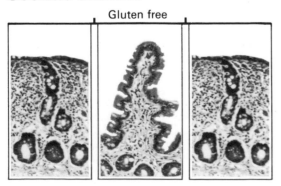

In Britain cystic fibrosis is the most common autosomal recessive disease in man. An abnormal gene is inherited from each parent, who is clinically normal, and the risk of a recurrence in each subsequent pregnancy is one in four. A high sweat sodium concentration is essential for making the diagnosis. If the infant presents with malabsorption due to pancreatic insufficiency vigorous prophylactic treatment of the lungs can be started at an early age and may prevent or limit the development of chronic lung disease. The extent of permanent lung damage determines the ultimate prognosis but 75% of children are now reaching at least the teenage years, probably as a result of more aggressive treatment in the early years. The relation between the high sweat sodium concentrations, preventable chronic lung disease, and pancreatic insufficiency is unknown. A method for antenatal diagnosis has recently been published but studies are still in progress on a reliable neonatal screening test. At present the most promising test is the blood immunoreactive trypsin level. Tests for the carrier state have recently become available for some families. The steatorrhoea is reduced by giving supplements of pancreatic extract. The use of a low fat diet is controversial. Vitamin supplements are given. Prevention of chronic lung disease depends on regular physiotherapy given by the parents with the liberal use of antibiotics. An antibiotic, usually flucloxacillin or erythromycin, is given during every upper respiratory tract infection and during the subsequent two weeks. Some authorities give a prophylactic antibiotic continuously during the first year of life.

Coeliac disease

Gluten free

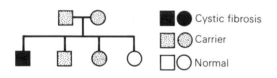

In coelic disease malabsorption is associated with a small intestinal mucosa which is completely flat on diagnosis, improves on a gluten-free diet, and relapses on challenge with gluten powder. There may be several years between the reintroduction of gluten and the recurrence of diarrhoea. The infants usually present between the ages of 5 and 7 months but may be seen for the first time at any age. Ideally the diagnosis should be confirmed by three jejunal biopsies and if it is proved a gluten-free diet is needed for life. Especially in children aged under 1 year, a flat jejunal biopsy can be found in other diseases such as gastroenteritis or cows' milk protein intolerance, and for this reason three biopsies are needed.

URINARY TRACT INFECTION

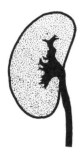

Each year about two children in each general practice and 300 in each health district have their first urinary tract infection. The ratio of girls to boys affected is about 2 to 1. Numerous studies have shown a radiological abnormality in 25–50% of these children. Vesicoureteric reflux is causally associated with pyelonephritis and renal scarring, which are responsible for 20% of the end stage renal failure in European patients below 40 years of age. Identification and treatment of children with reflux may prevent some cases of renal failure. Some children with urinary infection have surgically correctable abnormalities such as obstructive lesions or renal stones.

If severe renal scarring is present, which is rare, it has usually occurred by the age of 5 years. Therefore early diagnosis and effective treatment are especially important in this age group, but the symptoms may be insidious and the interpretation of routine specimens of urine difficult. The careful collection, handling and examination of urine specimens is crucial in avoiding unnecessary investigations.

Clinical features

Dysuria	Fever
Frequency	Vomiting
Abdominal pain	Lethargy
Enuresis	Slow gain in weight

There may be lethargy, vomiting, slow weight gain, fever, dysuria, frequency, abdominal pain, or bed wetting but sometimes only fever. Only about 20% of children with dysuria and frequency have a urinary infection. Girls with these symptoms often have vulvovaginitis (page 120). Frequency of micturition may be due to a behaviour problem rather than a urinary tract infection.

As the symptoms are not specific every ill child without a diagnosis as well as those with the features above must have a properly collected urine specimen examined for the presence of bacteria. This specimen must be taken before any antibiotics are given, and if the child is not dangerously ill it is preferable to withhold antibiotics until a specimen can be examined in the laboratory. If there is fever and pain in the loin admission to hospital is advisable as treatment is needed urgently to avoid possible renal damage. The urine should be routinely tested for glucose, but the presence of protein does not confirm a urinary tract infection or its absence exclude it.

Collection of urine

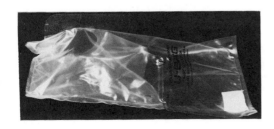

In infants a disposable adhesive plastic urinary bag is applied to the skin round the external genitalia after preliminary washing with water. The bag is removed as soon as a small amount of urine has been passed. A fresh mid-stream clean-catch specimen can often be obtained after gentle suprapubic stimulation by pressure or cold water, especially in boys. If the bag urine specimen contains more than 10×10^6 pus cells per litre or bacteria are seen in a fresh specimen or there is growth of more than 100×10^6 organisms per litre a further bag urine specimen should be taken, preferably after a bath, if the infant is not severely ill.

Urinary tract infection

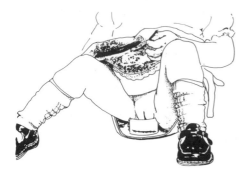

If the infant is ill or the second bag specimen is abnormal a further urine specimen may be obtained by suprapubic bladder puncture. Bacteria cultured from this specimen confirm a urinary tract infection.

A child who will sit on a potty or the lavatory seat can have a mid-stream specimen of urine collected, preferably after a bath. The growth of at least 100×10^6 bacteria per litre and the presence of the same organism with the same antibiotic sensitivities in three specimens of urine confirm the diagnosis.

Parents can be taught how to collect a mid-stream specimen of urine from a girl while she is sitting on a potty or the lavatory. As several specimens may be needed during the subsequent year time is well spent during the initial tuition. Special devices for collecting the mid-stream specimen have been devised using a removable tray.

Despite scrupulous care in the collection of urine by these methods it may be impossible to interpret the results of specimens obtained from some girls. A fine urinary catheter can be used to obtain a confirmatory specimen as several authorities no longer consider the procedure hazardous.

Laboratory examination of urine

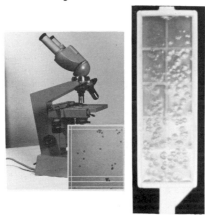

Microscopy for pus cells and culture should be performed within an hour of collection or the urine should be refrigerated at 4°C until examination is possible. Microscopy for pus or organisms is helpful in the sick child because it gives an immediate answer and is essential if any antibacterial drug has already been given as pus cells and organisms may be shown although the culture may be sterile.

An alternative is to use a dipslide to culture pathogens, and this method is useful in general practice.

Antibacterial treatment

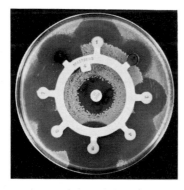

For most children treatment can await the results of bacterial sensitivity tests, but if immediate treatment is necessary co-trimoxazole is the drug of choice. The results of sensitivity tests to cultured pathogens will show whether a different drug is needed. The full therapeutic dose must be continued for 14 days and the urine should be cultured 3 and 10 days after the start of treatment to check that the infection has been eliminated. The urine should be sterile three days after the start of treatment. A high fluid intake will dilute the urinary bacterial count, stimulate frequent voiding, and ease dysuria.

Investigations

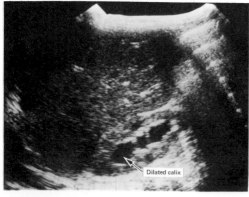

Infants less than a year should have an ultrasound examination of the renal tract, isotope renal scan, and cystourethrography. The isotope scan (^{99m}Tc dimercaptosuccinic acid (DMSA) scan) detects scars. Ultrasound shows obstructive lesions. Cystourethrography detects vesicoureteric reflux and should be performed under the protection of a suitable antibiotic. Intravenous urography (intravenous pyelogram) produces poor results in this age group.

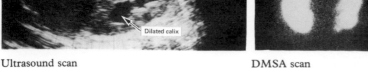
Dilated calix

Ultrasound scan

DMSA scan

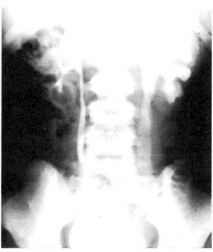
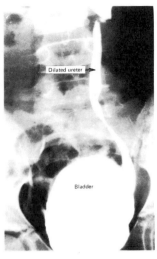
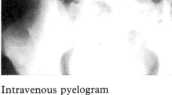

Intravenous pyelogram   Micturating cystogram

Children of 1 to 7 years should have either excretory urography or plain abdominal film, renal ultrasound, and DMSA scan. The excretory urography should be delayed for six weeks after the infection has been treated, while giving a prophylactic antibiotic, to allow the characteristic changes of scars to appear.

Children over 7 years have a plain abdominal film and renal ultrasound.

Micturating cystourethrogram should be performed in children over 1 year in the following groups:
(a) recurrence of infection;
(b) above studies are abnormal;
(c) fever and loin pain occurred in the first episode suggesting pyelonephritis;
(d) family history of chronic pyelonephritis.

Follow-up

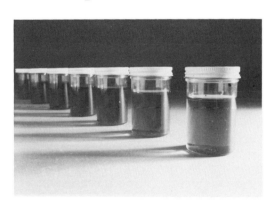

Regular urine cultures are advisable at monthly intervals initially and later at three monthly intervals as well as at times of fever or recurrence of symptoms. The urine should be cultured regularly while vesicoureteric reflux persists and in children with renal damage at least until the kidneys are fully grown (about the age of 16 years). The child's growth and blood pressure should be measured regularly.

If an anatomical abnormality is detected radiologically or if infections recur the radiological investigations may need to be repeated to determine whether renal growth is normal and whether there is evidence of fresh scarring. The intervals of these investigations vary with the problem, and excessive radiation can be avoided by consulting a paediatrician.

Continuous prophylaxis

Vesicouretic reflux

Recurrent symptomatic infection

Renal damage

The object of prophylaxis is to prevent reinfection of a susceptible urinary tract after bacteriuria has been eliminated. Prophylaxis should be used in children with vesicoureteric reflux, those with recurrent symptomatic infection, and children with renal damage until the kidneys are fully grown. The ideal drug should be absorbed high in the alimentary tract, be excreted in high concentration in the urine, and not cause resistance in the flora of the lower bowel. Co-trimoxazole and nitrofurantoin fulfil these criteria, and a single daily dose of about half the standard 24-hour dose should be given in the evening. Nitrofurantoin has the disadvantage that it often causes nausea and vomiting even at this low dose. These patients are best managed at a special urinary tract infection clinic at the local district hospital.

ENURESIS

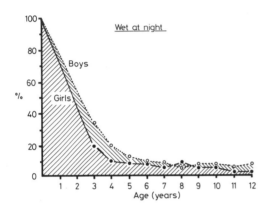

Wetting the bed is normal at birth, a nuisance at 5 years, and then it becomes increasingly disturbing for both child and mother. Siblings who share the same room or bed and the father whose living room is dominated by wet sheets resent the problem. Ten per cent of children still wet the bed at the age of 5 and 14% of these become dry each succeeding year. The electric enuresis alarm (buzzer) is an effective aid but an enthusiastic teacher of the use of the alarm contributes to its success.

History

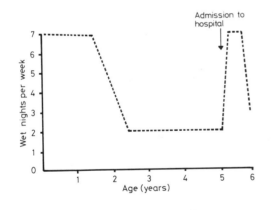

The mother should be asked what is the longest period that the child has been dry at night. If he has been dry for a least two nights in succession there is likely to be no structural abnormality. If the enuresis started after a long period of dryness a precipitating event should be sought. Ten per cent of children with enuresis also wet themselves during the day, and this does not alter the diagnosis or management.

A urinary tract infection may cause frequency of micturition and enuresis while a poor stream in boys suggests an abnormality of the urinary tract. A neurological abnormality severe enough to cause bladder problems will usually interfere with walking.

The reason for referral at a particular time rather than earlier may indicate the need for treatment. The child may be motivated to change—for example, because he wants to go to a camp.

Enuresis to a late age in one of the parents suggests a familial pattern. Delay in other aspects of development may show that the child has other abnormalities. Common precipitating factors are the birth of a brother or sister, marital discord, admission to hospital, maternal illness, or moving home.

Examination

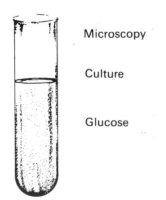

Enlarged kidneys or bladder and midline naevi or other markers of spinal abnormality should be sought. The reflexes at the ankles, gait, and sensation over the sacral area should be examined. In every case a sample of urine must be sent to the laboratory to exclude infection, and glycosuria can be excluded by a Diastix test. Unless there is a specific indication other than enuresis an intravenous pyelogram should not be performed.

Treatment

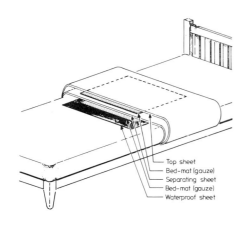

	1st Week	2nd Week	3rd Week	4th Week	
Monday		★		★	
Tuesday			★	★	
Wednesday	★		★	★	
Thursday		★	★	★	
Friday				★	
Saturday		★	★	★	
Sunday	★			★	

No treatment is indicated for a child under the age of $4\frac{1}{2}$ years. Ideally the parents and child should be seen together at first and then the child separately. The child should be given an opportunity to explain what he feels and to be shown that he is the patient and that his cooperation is necessary for success.

Fluid restriction is not helpful. Charts with stars provide a method whereby the child keeps records himself. Young children enjoy filling the spaces, and the recording of dry nights should be emphasised. Some children become completely dry after using a chart for a few weeks without any other treatment. On the other hand, some paediatricians find that this method is very disheartening to the child who is not successful.

Lifting the child on to a potty before the parents go to sleep is sometimes associated with a dry bed in the morning. This treatment can be used until a decision is made to use a buzzer.

Buzzer treatment

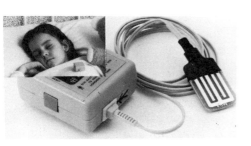

Top sheet
Bed-mat (gauze)
Separating sheet
Bed-mat (gauze)
Waterproof sheet

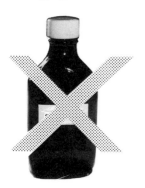

Children over the age of 6 use the alarm easily but it can be successful at the age of 5. Whether the child sleeps in his own bed and in his own room will determine whether a standard buzzer can be used. Temporary changes in sleeping arrangements may be necessary to prevent others in the room being woken by the buzzer. A special alarm which vibrates the pillow can be used where sleeping arrangements cannot be changed and for children who do not wake when the buzzer sounds.

Hospitals, health centres, and local health clinics have stocks of alarms, but expert advice on the use of the buzzer is needed from a committed person. This could be a doctor, nurse, or health visitor. The child and mother must be shown how to arrange the alarm in the bed and how to test it.

There are three types of detector, each of which is attached to an alarm. A new type of sensor is attached to the child's pants. The older types of detector consist of single or paired mats. The child sleeps on a sheet which separates him from a detector—a metal mat—connected to an alarm buzzer. Urine completes the circuit. The alarm wakens the child, who stops the urine stream, gets out of bed, turns off the alarm, and goes to the lavatory. The amount of urine passed before the child wakes becomes progressively smaller and he either wakes before the alarm starts or he sleeps throughout the night without passing urine. The child should be seen a week after issuing the alarm and then at longer intervals. After he has been dry for six consecutive weeks the alarm is removed from the bed but kept at home ready for use if necessary for a further six weeks. About 80% of the children become dry within four months and most within the first two months of treatment. About 10% of children relapse but respond quickly to a second course of treatment with the alarm.

Five to 20% of children will still be wetting the bed after four months' treatment and these should be given a respite of a year before using the alarm again.

Drugs and psychiatrists

Tricyclic antidepressants have been used successfully in enuresis but there is a high relapse rate when the drug is stopped. A disadvantage of this treatment is that the pleasant-tasting medicine has caused severe side effects and death through children taking overdoses. These drugs cannot be recommended.

When enuresis is a part of an emotional disorder the child should be referred to a child psychiatrist. Chronic constipation or the passage of formed stools in inappropriate places may occur with enuresis in a severely disturbed child. Enuresis starting after a long period of dry nights suggests a precipitating cause—for example, separation of parents. If buzzer treatment has failed, the possibility of an underlying emotional cause should be sought.

SYSTOLIC MURMURS

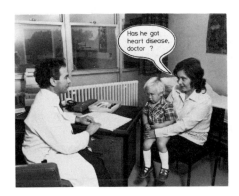

Congenital heart disease occurs in about one in every 100 live births but the commonest clinical problem is the child with a murmur discovered during a routine examination or during an acute illness. Most of these children have no cardiac disease.

The minority with physical disease usually have a ventricular septal defect or mild pulmonary stenosis. Most of the ventricular septal defects close spontaneously before the child reaches the age of 5 years.

Loud murmurs are always due to cardiac disease. Soft murmurs may be either caused by cardiac disease or have no pathological significance (benign or innocent murmurs).

Loud systolic murmurs

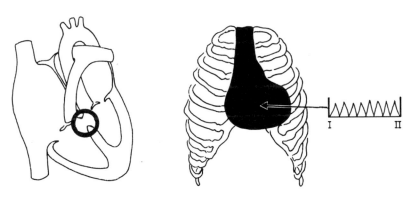

Ventricular septal defect is the most common congenital heart disease in childhood. It produces a loud murmur maximal in the fourth left intercostal space close to the sternum. Although it is maximal at that site it radiates in all directions and may be heard as high as the clavicle.

Pulmonary stenosis causes a loud systolic murmur maximal in the pulmonary area, which is conducted to the left lung posteriorly.

Aortic stenosis produces a murmur which may be maximal to the right of the upper sternum and to the left of the midsternum and is well conducted to both sides of the neck.

Soft systolic murmurs due to organic disease

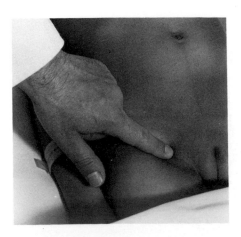

Atrial septal defect causes a soft systolic murmur in the pulmonary area due to the increased flow of blood through the pulmonary valve. This lesion is often first noted in adult life, when the symptoms appear. In atrial septal defect the second heart sound is widely split and does not vary with respiration. In contrast, in normal children the second heart sound is widely split in inspiration and less in expiration.

Children with coarctation of the aorta often have a short systolic murmur heard over the back between the scapulae. The diagnosis is not missed if the femoral arteries are palpated routinely. Children with coarctation of the aorta often have other lesions, such as aortic stenosis, and the finding of a murmur due to that lesion may bring the coarctation to light.

Differential diagnosis

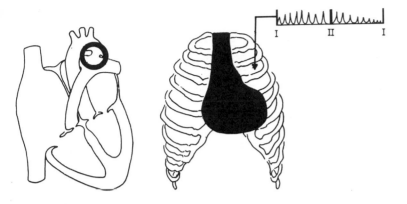

For those who are not cardiologists systolic murmurs which spill over into diastole may be difficult to differentiate from purely systolic murmurs. There are two important examples: *patent ductus arteriosus* and the *venous hum*. Most children with persistent patent ductus arteriosus have no symptoms. The murmur is maximal in the second left intercostal space lateral to the pulmonary area. The murmur may radiate down the left sternal edge and to the apex. The murmur is described as sounding like machinery. High volume pulses are present when the ductus is widely patent. Other types of congenital heart disease, particularly ventricular septal defect, may also be present.

The venous hum is a continuous murmur throughout systole and diastole and is heard best under the inner end of the right clavicle with the child sitting up. It can be abolished by lying the child down. It is a normal finding.

Soft systolic murmurs of benign origin

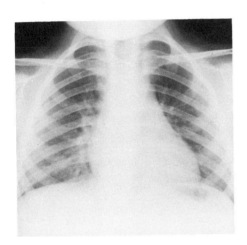

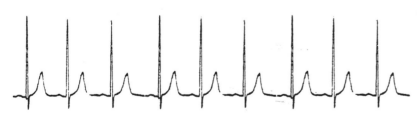

Benign systolic murmurs are soft, short, and low pitched. They are heard maximally to the left of the sternum. The murmur becomes louder when the patient lies down and softer when he stands up. Organic disease is usually excluded by the character of the murmur and the absence of any symptoms or abnormal signs in the cardiovascular system. The femoral pulses must be checked. A normal chest radiograph and electrocardiogram may help to confirm the diagnosis but where the diagnosis is still uncertain the opinion of a paediatric cardiologist and echocardiography may be helpful.

Fever or anaemia intensify benign murmurs and a murmur that sounded loud at the time of an acute illness may be almost inaudible in an outpatient clinic a few weeks later. Anaemia may be difficult to diagnose clinically and a haemoglobin estimation is advisable.

Benign murmurs: discussion with parents

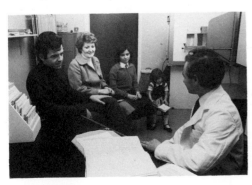

Benign or innocent murmurs do not indicate heart disease and need no treatment. Many parents fail to understand what the murmur means despite careful explanation, and unnecessary fear and anxiety is generated. Despite reassurances by a doctor the parents may restrict the physical activities of the child, to his detriment. The parents may misinterpret what is told to them and believe that their child *has* heart disease.

Systolic murmurs

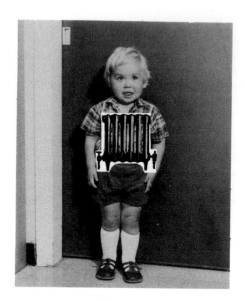

If the murmur is discovered during a routine examination and the doctor is convinced that it is benign there is no advantage in discussing it with the parents. On the other hand, if there is a doubt about the nature of the murmur the parents must be told that the child has a murmur. If the murmur has been noted on one occasion it is likely to be heard again at routine examinations and whenever the child has a fever. If the child is acutely ill with a high fever and the mother is very anxious it may be better to postpone telling her about the murmur until the child has been examined in the convalescent period. If there is a possibility that another doctor will see the child at that time it may be better to discuss it at the first visit and avoid the possibility that it will be forgotten.

When the murmur is being discussed, preferably in the presence of both parents, it should be emphasised that it is a normal sound heard in children with normal hearts; that the noise is probably due to blood flowing through the tubes, and in some cases more noise is produced than in others, similar to the noise in some central heating systems. Doctors initially have to exclude disease but when they have done that the child should be considered completely normal and should be treated as a normal child. Ample opportunity must be given to allow the parents to ask questions to enable them to understand this difficult concept.

GROWTH FAILURE

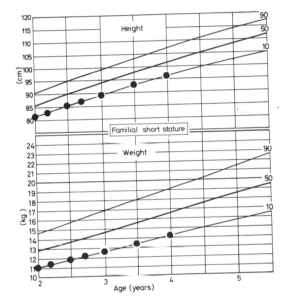

Parents may be worried because they consider their child to be too short, or too thin, or both. The infant's height is usually not noticed until he starts walking and is compared with his contemporaries. This coincides with the period of negativism and a normal reduction in appetite and food intake. Most children whose parents seek advice have familial short stature but the rest have a wide variety of problems, some of which can be improved after an accurate diagnosis has been made. This chapter is concerned mainly with growth after the age of 1 year but some aspects of earlier growth have been included to put the topic into perspective.

Growth is a dynamic process and more than one accurate measurement is needed to assess it. Infants under 1 year are weighed naked, but over 1 year children wear vest and pants only. Weight can be measured accurately with minimal skill and cheap equipment. This allows any deviations from normal to be detected within a few weeks during the time of rapid growth—that is, during the first few months of life. Another index is needed for comparison, and until the age of 2 years the head circumference is reliable. After the age of 1 year standing height can be measured, but a precision stadiometer and attention to detail is needed to provide reproducible results. The head must be held with the external auditory meatus and the outer angle of the eye in the same horizontal plane and gentle upward traction applied to the mastoid processes. Two measurements six months apart must be made before the rate of growth can be confidently assessed.

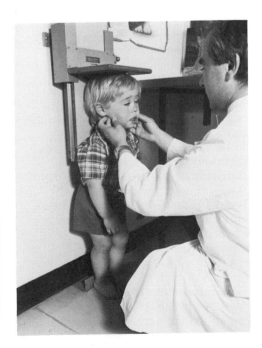
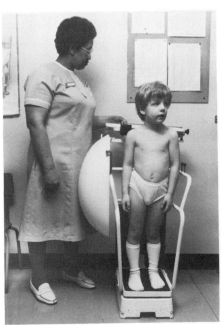
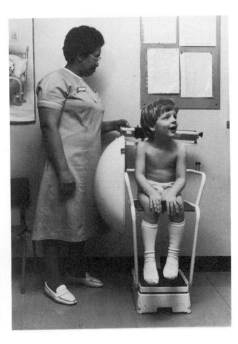

Growth failure

Too thin or too light

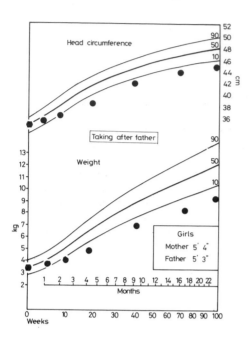

A child is usually on a similar centile for weight, head circumference, and height. Children of tall parents tend to be towards the 90th centile and those of short parents near the 10th centile. Most children remain on the same centiles for the rest of their lives. Plotting these measurements on a chart in routine clinics helps to confirm that the child is receiving adequate food and is growing normally. Although birth weight depends mainly on maternal size, some children are more similar to one parent than the other in final size. By the age of 1 year these adjustments have usually been made. If only their weights are recorded children may appear to be either failing to thrive if the father is small or gaining weight excessively if the father is tall. If height and head circumference are plotted as well the series of measurements can be seen to be parallel.

The child who is abnormally thin has lost subcutaneous fat, which is shown by wasting of the buttocks and the inner aspects of the thighs. The growth chart then shows a weight which is on a centile considerably lower than that of the head circumference or height. A child from a family of a narrow body build may show a similar pattern if he is measured only once. But there will be no clinical signs of wasting, and if the measurements are repeated after an interval the increase in weight will parallel that in height or head circumference.

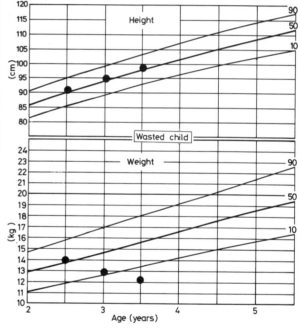

Familial patterns of growth

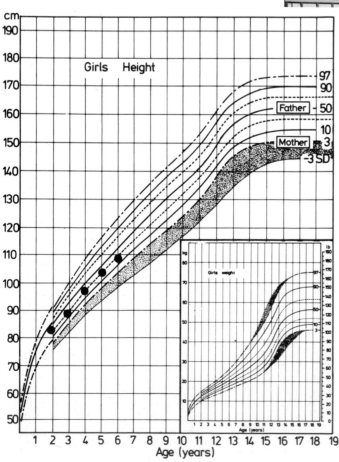

Most children have a height approximately midway between those of their parents when an adjustment for sex has been made. For boys 13 cm should be added to the sum of the parents' heights and for girls this should be subtracted. Division of this total by two gives the expected adult height for that child. Alternatively the height centile for each parent can be determined from the chart which ends at 19 years, and the child usually has a centile between the two values.

A child with familial short stature will follow the growth pattern of both or one of his parents or another close relative but the diagnosis needs to be confirmed by checking that he is growing at a normal rate—that is, 5 cm or more per year.

Normal rate but atypical patterns of growth

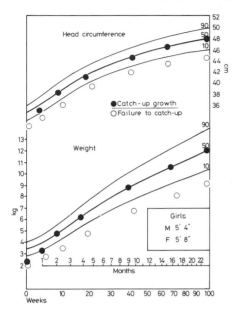

Most infants who grow poorly before birth have a period of "catch-up" growth during the first few months of life. A few, however, continue to grow at the same rate after birth. Although they are short their body proportions are normal but they never reach the normal range for height and weight.

Some short schoolchildren have a family history of similar delay in growth and development, and during the school years the height and bone age are usually retarded. These children may become very distressed towards puberty when they realise that they are not growing as fast as their friends who have a prepubertal growth spurt before them.

Deficient food or malabsorption

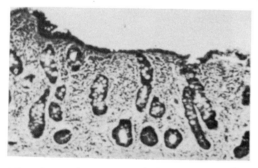

Malnutrition from lack of food probably occurs in some of the lower socioeconomic classes in affluent countries as well as in developing countries. Unrecognised poor lactation is becoming more prominent as the incidence of breast-feeding increases. Psychosocial deprivation may decrease the amount of food eaten but is often associated with temporary growth hormone deficiency. Cystic fibrosis and coeliac disease are the most common causes of severe malabsorption, though only one in 2000 children is affected by each of these diseases.

Endocrine problems and other disorders

Children with hypothyroidism may have no distinctive clinical features, and the diagnosis is often delayed. Girls with congenital adrenal hyperplasia are virilised. Growth hormone deficiency should be suspected if the child is extremely short and is below the −3SD line on the height chart.

If previous measurements are not available he should be measured again six months later. If his growth curve is not on or parallel to a centile line or he has grown only 3 cm or less he should be referred to a paediatrician.

The mechanism whereby patients with cerebral palsy, uraemia, chronic heart failure, and liver disease fail to grow well is complex, but most of these children have a poor appetite and are likely to have a deficient food intake.

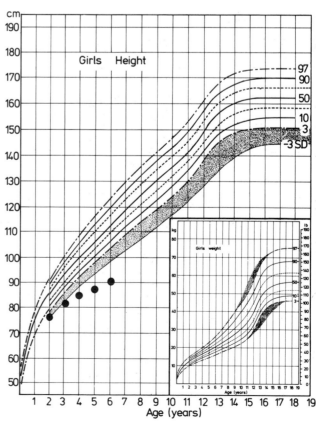

Growth failure

Deficient growth potential of bones

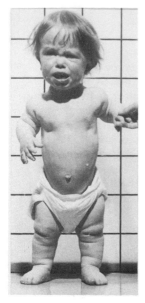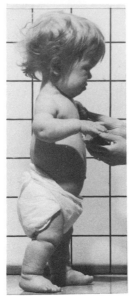

Infants with obvious bone disease such as achondroplasia as well as other children with named syndromes can be recognised by their abnormal appearance and the systems affected. Girls with Turner's syndrome may have no gross abnormalities on physical examination, and leucocyte chromosome studies are needed to exclude this diagnosis.

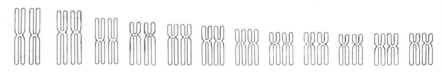

Referral to hospital

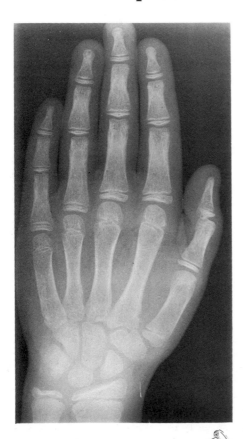

If the child's low height centile is similar to that of a parent or close relative and he had no symptoms or abnormal signs familial short stature can be diagnosed. This should be confirmed by measuring him again six months later and showing that he is growing on a line which is parallel to the third centile—that is, at a normal rate.

Children with any of the following features should be referred to hospital for further investigation.
(1) Clinical signs of wasting.
(2) Symptoms such as dyspnoea on exercise or chronic diarrhoea.
(3) Abnormal appearance or signs of disease such as congenital heart disease.
(4) Documented evidence of a slow rate of growth (3 cm or less) detected by two measurements six months apart.
(5) Height below the -3SD line on the growth chart.
(6) Social problems or deprivation. About a third of children below the third centile who have no physical disease come from severely deprived backgrounds and are not only stunted physically but also retarded in tests of intellectual function. Some of these children are suffering from neglect.

Patients seen in hospital will have their height and weight measured carefully. A radiograph of the left hand is taken to measure the bone age and blood is taken to estimate haemoglobin, plasma thyroxine, thyrotrophin, and urea concentrations. Girls with documented slow growth have blood taken for chromosomal analysis. A sweat test for cystic fibrosis is performed and jejunal biopsy considered. A test for growth hormone after stimulation is performed last because some of the previous conditions may cause confusingly low levels and many paediatricians prefer to estimate the growth rate first.

Haemoglobin
ESR
Thyroxine
Urea
Chromosomes (girls only)

COMMON RASHES

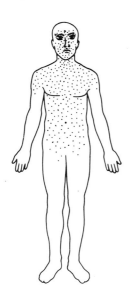

Rashes usually occur as part of one of the common infectious diseases of childhood, but these must be distinguished from dermatological causes. The characteristics of the lesions, distribution, changes with time, and accompanying features help to determine the diagnosis. A previous attack of an infectious disease makes a further attack unlikely, but a high incidence of wrong diagnoses of some rashes, particularly the misdiagnosis of rashes as being caused by rubella, detracts from the value of this history.

Purpura

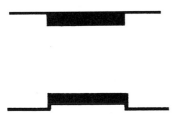

Purpuric lesions are caused by haemorrhages in the skin and they do not disappear on pressure. The child with purpura usually needs to be admitted immediately as he may have meningococcal septicaemia, leukaemia, or idiopathic thrombocytopenic purpura. Henoch–Schönlein purpura is more common than these conditions, however, and is distributed over the extensor surfaces of the limbs as well as the buttocks, and some of the purpuric lesions are raised. If the rash has all the characteristic features of Henoch–Schönlein purpura admission is not needed.

Macules and papules

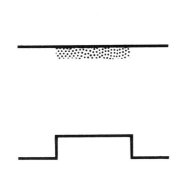

Macules are discrete lesions that change the colour of the skin, though they fade on pressure. They may be of any size or shape and may be pink or red.

Discrete pink minute macules occur in rubella, when they are accompanied by suboccipital lymphadenopathy. In both roseola and rubella suboccipital lymphadenopathy is pronounced, but in roseola the appearance of the rash coincides with the disappearance of all other symptoms. The child with rubella may have slight fever. In contrast infants with roseola have high fever and irritability for three or four days before the macular rash appears. Despite the high fever the child may play normally.

Papules are solid palpable projections above the surface of the skin. Insect bites are one cause of these lesions, which are called papular urticaria.

Common rashes

Maculopapular rash

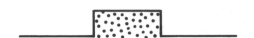

A maculopapular rash is a mixture of the two types of lesion described above, which tend to be confluent. A maculopapular rash is the typical rash of measles, when it is always accompanied by cough and sometimes by nasal discharge. The most common problem is to distinguish measles from a drug rash, which may itch. Koplik spots have usually disappeared by this stage, but if they persist they may be helpful. The drug may have been given for an upper respiratory tract infection and the clinical picture may mimic measles.

A maculopapular rash occurs in glandular fever, especially in patients who have received ampicillin or one of its derivatives. Patients who have been receiving ampicillin may suffer a drug rash during their first course of treatment. The rash usually occurs about the 10th day after starting the drug. Usually a second exposure after an interval is needed for a drug rash to occur.

Vesicles

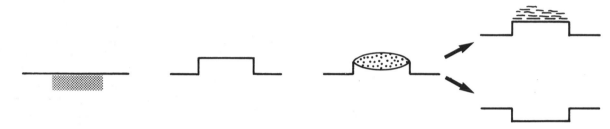

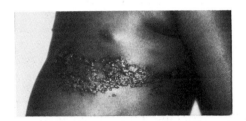

Vesicles are blisters caused by fluid raising the horny layer of the epidermis. In chickenpox the lesions pass through the stages of macule, papule, and vesicle within two days and crops of rash occur. A fairly clear vesicle on the skin is the diagnostic lesion. Vesicles change to pustules and later to scales or ulcers.

In herpes zoster a rash occurs in the distribution of a sensory nerve. Itching may occur before the rash appears.

An infant's first contact with herpes simplex virus may cause vesicles and severe ulcers in the mouth or on the vulva or conjunctiva.

Summer outbreaks of hand, foot, and mouth disease are recognised by the pearly white vesicles at these sites, which are due to a Coxsackie virus.

Wheals

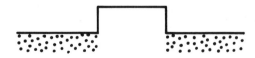

Wheals are raised lesions with a pale centre surrounded by a red area. The rash is accompanied by itching, and the cause is usually not discovered. The rash may be difficult to diagnose in the resolving phase.

Desquamation

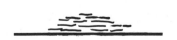

Desquamation is a loss of epidermal cells which produces a "scaly" eruption. Desquamation is found in atopic eczema and affects the flexures, face, and neck but may be more widespread. Psoriasis produces round scaly lesions 0.5–1 cm in diameter on the face, trunk, and limbs.

INFECTIOUS DISEASES

Measles

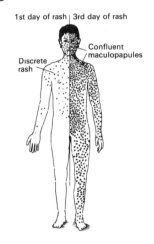

1st day of rash | 3rd day of rash

Confluent maculopapules

Discrete rash

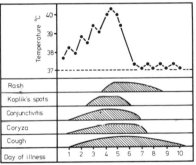

After an incubation period of 10–14 days there is a prodromal illness with cough, fever, and nasal discharge. The presence of a cough is essential for the diagnosis. During the prodromal period there are minute white spots on a red background on the buccal mucosa opposite the molar teeth (Koplik's spots). After about four days a maculopapular rash appears on the face and behind the ears and spreads downwards to cover the whole body while older lesions become more blotchy. As the rash appears the Koplik's spots fade. The rash begins to fade after three or four days and is accompanied by a fall in the temperature and reduction in malaise. Some children become irritable. Measles is not contagious after the fifth day of the rash, but exposure has usually occurred before the diagnosis is obvious. Attempts to isolate siblings from each other are useless.

Acute otitis media is the commonest complication of measles; signs usually appear about three days after the onset of the rash. Antibiotics should be given if these signs appear but there is no place for prophylactic antibiotics against otitis media. The onset of bronchopneumonia may be difficult to detect as a severe cough is part of the measles. A raised respiratory rate at rest or adventitious sounds are confirmatory signs. The serious complication of encephalitis occurs in about 1 in 1000 affected children and causes drowsiness, vomiting, headache, and convulsions about seven days after the onset of measles. In developing countries measles has a high morbidity and mortality, and diarrhoea is a common feature, particularly in severely malnourished children.

A drug reaction in the presence of a viral infection is difficult to distinguish from measles rash. Features suggesting a drug reaction are lack of cough, an irritating rash, or an atypical distribution of spots.

Rubella

1st day of rash | 3rd day of rash

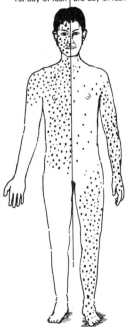

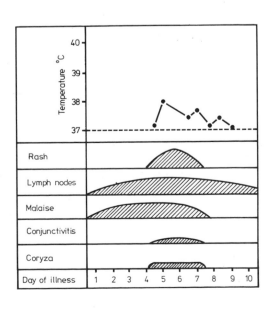

Rubella or German measles is usually a mild illness and the rash may not be noticed. The incidence of rubella infections without rash may be 25%. When a rash does occur it appears as a pink, minute, discrete, macular rash on the face and trunk after an incubation period of 14–21 days. The suboccipital lymph nodes are enlarged and there may be generalised lymphadenopathy. Thrombocytopenia, encephalitis, and arthritis are rare complications of rubella. The period of infectivity probably extends from the latter part of the incubation period to the end of the first week of the rash.

If rubella occurs during the first five months of pregnancy the fetus may die or develop congenital heart disease, mental retardation, deafness, or cataracts. If *any rash* occurs during pregnancy a specimen of blood should be taken immediately and again 10 days later for measuring rubella antibody titres to determine whether a recent infection with rubella has occurred. If there has been previous serological evidence that the mother is immune to rubella no tests are required.

Infectious diseases

Roseola

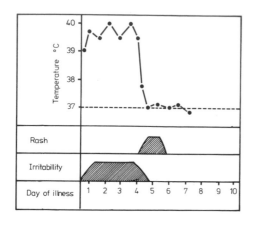

Although fever may be present in the prodromal period of any infectious disease of childhood, pronounced fever is a notorious feature of roseola infantum. There may be a convulsion at the onset. The temperature usually reaches 39°C to 40°C and remains at this level for about three days. The temperature falls and the child becomes well as discrete minute pink macules appear on the trunk; these may spread to the limbs within a few hours. The child appears less ill than might be expected from the height of the fever. The suboccipital, cervical, and postauricular lymph nodes are often enlarged and there is often neutropenia.

Chickenpox

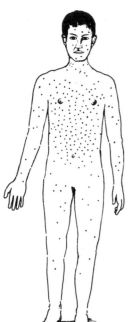

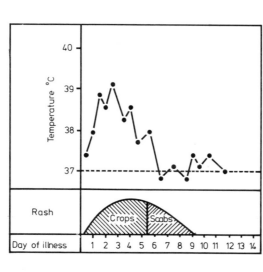

After an incubation period of 14–17 days the rash appears on the trunk and face. The spots appear in crops passing from macule to papule, vesicle, and pustule within two days. Lesions in the mouth produce painful shallow ulcers and if they are in the trachea and bronchi may produce a severe cough. Severe irritation of the skin may occur and may be alleviated by calamine lotion and oral promethazine. The lesions normally pass through a pustular stage, and as this is not bacterial in origin, local or oral antibiotics are rarely required. Encephalitis is rare but often produces cerebellar signs with ataxia. This occurs three to eight days after the onset of the rash, and most patients recover completely.

Secondarily infected lesions and scabs removed by scratching may be followed by scarring. A child with chickenpox may transmit the disease to other susceptible children from one day before the onset of the rash until all the vesicles have crusted. The dry scabs do not contain active virus. Complete crusting of the lesions occurs from 5 to 10 days after onset. Chickenpox may be contracted from a patient with herpes zoster.

Scarlet fever

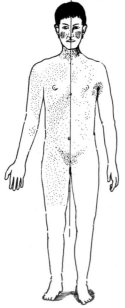

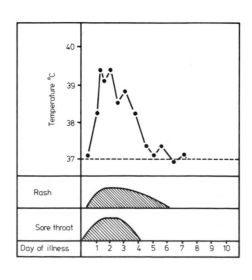

Scarlet fever is less virulent than it was 40 years ago. Sequelae such as rheumatic fever and acute glomerulonephritis are very rare. It is caused by an erythrogenic strain of group A haemolytic streptococci. After an incubation period of two to four days fever, headache, and tonsillitis appear. Pin-point macules which blanch on pressure occur on the trunk and neck with increased density in the neck, axillae, and groins. A thick white coating on the tongue peels on the third day, leaving a "strawberry" appearance. The rash lasts about six days and is followed by peeling. A 10-day course of oral penicillin eradicates the organism and may prevent other children from being infected.

WHOOPING COUGH

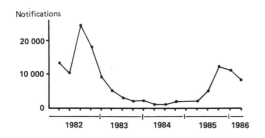

Notifications

The present high incidence of whooping cough warrants a reappraisal of prevention and management. Young infants receive no protective immunity from their mothers and have the highest incidence of complications. Immunisation is directed at increasing herd immunity and reducing exposure of infants to the disease in older children. Persistent neurological abnormalities associated with immunisation occur, particularly when the known contraindications are ignored or not elicited.

Risks

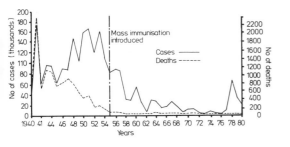

Risk of dying from: *

Smoking (10 cigarettes /day)	1/400
All accidents	1/2000
Traffic accidents	1/8000
Leukaemia from natural causes	1/20 000
Work in industry	1/30 000
Drowning	1/30 000
Poisoning	1/100 000
Natural disasters	1/500 000
Rock climbing for 90 seconds	1/1 000 000
Driving 50 miles	1/1 000 000
Being struck by lightning	1/2 000 000
Risk of persistent neurological damage from full course of pertussis vaccination	1/100 000

* From the Royal Commission on environmental pollution.   Sixth report.

The National Childhood Encephalopathy Study showed that the incidence of serious neurological illnesses in immunised children was slightly but significantly higher than in unimmunised children of the same age seven days after immunisation, particularly in the first 72 hours. No such excess occurred after diphtheria and tetanus immunisation without pertussis. Normal children undergoing a full course of triple vaccination have a risk of about 1 in 100 000 of suffering persistent neurological damage. The Meade Panel, which studied the same problem for 1970–4 retrospectively without control data, suggested that the incidence of persistent brain damage in normal children was about 1 in 155 000 injections or about 1 in 53 000 children; 49% of children with neurological problems after triple vaccine had at least one contraindication to immunisation.

The acceptance rates for pertussis immunisation in England and Wales fell from 79% in 1973 to 31% in 1978. From 1977 to 1979 notifications of pertussis were higher than the rate in any epidemic in the previous 20 years. The attack rate was especially high where immunisation rates were lowest. Since 1977 the incidence of pertussis has remained constantly above the previous levels, with additional peaks. The vaccine modified infectivity within a family so that 2 out of 10 vaccinated siblings compared with 7 out of 10 unvaccinated siblings contracted the disease. Immunised children also seemed to have a milder illness. In 1977–80 there were 28 deaths from whooping cough in England and Wales compared with two deaths in children who developed a neurological illness within 7 days of immunisation in the three years of the National Encephalopathy Study. During the 1977–9 epidemic there were about 5000 admissions to hospital, 200 cases of pneumonia, and 83 cases of convulsions related to whooping cough. Recent studies in London have shown that lung function returns to normal after whooping cough.

Whooping cough

Contraindications to immunisation

Is the baby unwell in any way?   YES/NO
Has the baby had any side effects from previous immunisations?   YES/NO
Did the baby behave normally during the first week of life?   YES/NO
Has the baby, or anyone in the immediate family, ever had fits or convulsions?   YES/NO
Is the baby developing normally?   YES/NO

Mothers can fill out a card in the waiting room at each visit for immunisation.

According to the advice from the Joint Committee on Vaccination and Immunisation, the contraindications to whooping cough immunisation are: a reaction to a preceding dose, cerebral irritation in the neonatal period, and fits. Immunisation is not absolutely contraindicated in children whose parents or siblings have a history of idiopathic epilepsy, those with developmental delay due to a neurological defect, or those with neurological disease, but individual cases need careful assessment. The risk of damage from immunisation is higher than normal in these children, but so is the risk of severe effects of whooping cough. A personal or family history of allergy is no longer thought to be a contraindication, but doctors should use their discretion in each case. If an infant has an acute febrile illness immunisation is best postponed, but minor infections without fever or systemic upset are not contraindications.

Diagnosis

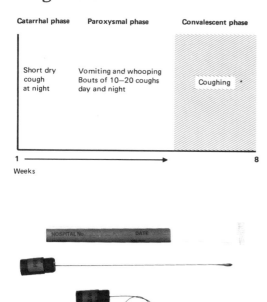

Catarrhal phase	Paroxysmal phase	Convalescent phase
Short dry cough at night	Vomiting and whooping Bouts of 10–20 coughs day and night	Coughing

1 — 8
Weeks

Whooping cough is difficult to diagnose during the first 7 to 14 days of the illness (catarrhal phase), when there is a short dry, nocturnal cough. Later, bouts of 10–20 short dry coughs occur day and night; each is on the same high note or rises in pitch. A long attack of coughing is followed by a sharp indrawing of breath, which may produce the crowing sound, or whoop. Some children, especially babies, with *Bordetella pertussis* infection never develop the whoop. Feeding with crumbly food often provokes a coughing spasm, which may culminate in vomiting. Afterwards there is a short period when the child can be fed again without provoking coughing. In uncomplicated cases there are no abnormal respiratory signs.

The most important differential diagnosis in infants is bronchiolitis; this is usually due to the respiratory syncytial virus, which produces epidemics of winter cough in infants under 1 year. For the first few days there may be only bouts of vibratory rasping cough which never produce a whoop. Later rhonchi or crepitations are heard in the chest and the infant either deteriorates or improves rapidly within a few days. Older siblings infected with the virus may have a milder illness. Other viruses may cause acute bronchitis with coughing but there are seldom more than two coughs at a time.

A properly taken pernasal swab plated promptly on a specific medium should reveal *Bordetella pertussis* in most patients during the first few weeks of the illness. A blood lymphocyte count of $10 \times 10^9/1$ or more with a normal erythrocyte sedimentation rate suggests whooping cough.

Management

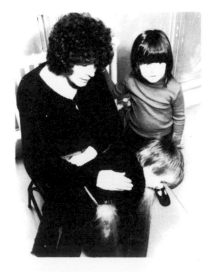

If the diagnosis is suspected in the catarrhal phase (usually because a sibling has had recognisable whooping cough) a 10-day course of erythromycin may be given to the child and to other children in the home. Parents must be warned that an antibiotic may shorten the course of the disease only in the early stages and is unlikely to affect established illness. Vomiting can be treated by giving soft, not crumbly, food or small amounts of fluid hourly.

No medicine reliably improves the cough. Salbutamol has been used in a dosage of 0.3 mg/kg/24 hours divided into three doses. When sleep is disturbed some authorities recommend that the child should be given a bedtime dose of 3–5 mg/kg of phenobarbitone or a large dose of promethazine hydrochloride starting with 1 mg/kg. In severe cases mothers can be taught to give physiotherapy, which may help to clear secretions, especially before the infant goes to sleep. An attack may be stopped by a gentle slap on the back.

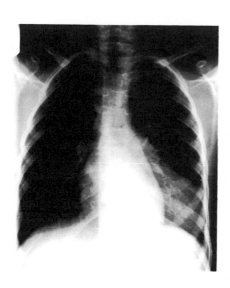

The threshold for admission should be lower for children aged under 6 months. Convulsions and cyanosis during coughing attacks are absolute indications for admission to an isolation cubicle. Parents often become exhausted by sleep loss, and arranging for different members of the family to sleep with the child will give the mother a respite. The cough usually lasts for 8 to 12 weeks and may recur when the child has any new viral respiratory infection during the subsequent year. If the child is generally ill or the cough has not improved after six weeks a chest radiograph should be performed to exclude bronchopneumonia or lobar collapse, which need treatment with physiotherapy and antibiotics. Long-term effects on the lung, such as bronchiectasis, are rare in developed countries.

The infant will not be infective for other children after about four weeks from the beginning of the illness or about two days after erythromycin is started. The incubation period is about seven days and contacts who have no symptoms two weeks after exposure have usually escaped infection.

PAEDIATRIC DERMATOLOGY

Atopic eczema

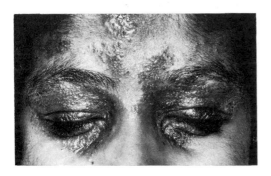

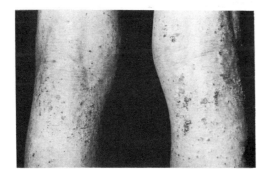

Atopic eczema affects about 5% of the population. Some 70% of patients have a family history of atopy, shown by eczema, asthma, or hay fever. Atopic eczema is characterised by itching and red vesicular patches with a marked predilection for the face and the flexures. A remission often occurs between 2 and 4 years but may be shortlived, and recurrence in childhood may be severe and cause gradual lichenification of the skin with greater involvement of the hands and feet. Atopic children have a lower threshold to pruritic stimuli, and some children are worse during the cold weather and others when it is hot and humid. Woollen clothing also irritates atopic skin. Dietary restriction is controversial and in our experience of very limited value. It should only be considered in children with severe atopic eczema who do not respond adequately to topical therapy.

In infants and small children the itching, the anxiety caused by it, and the social stigma of atopic eczema allow little opportunity for experimentation with unpleasant medications of uncertain effect. Acute eczema, which is nearly always secondarily infected, should be treated with a potent topical steroid–antibiotic combination and a systemic antibiotic. Often there are no obvious signs of infection. Fluorinated steroids should not be applied to the face for prolonged periods as atrophy of the skin may occur. When the acute phase has passed, usually within 10 days, a weaker topical steroid without antibiotic is used. Patients should be advised to avoid medicated soap, though a superfatted soap may be used with lubricants which help to moisten and soften the skin (e.g. aqueous cream, Unguentum Merck). These are best applied to wet skin at the end of the bath. Nocturnal itching can be diminished with an antihistamine, such as trimeprazine tartrate or hydroxyzine hydrochloride.

Eczema herpeticum

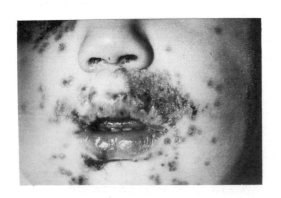

Herpes simplex infection, often primary, may complicate active or resolving atopic eczema. Kaposi's varicelliform eruption is a rapidly forming vesicular eruption which occurs mainly on abnormal skin but can become generalised. Fever and lymphadenopathy are usually present and there may be ocular and neurological complications. Patients should be isolated and receive antibiotics to prevent secondary bacterial infection. In addition acyclovir (Zovirax), an antiviral agent effective *in vitro* against herpes simplex virus, is prescribed for topical use and may also be required intravenously if the infection is severe or if there are neurological complications. Steroids, both topical and systemic, should be avoided though pre-existing systemic steroid treatment should not be stopped suddenly.

Impetigo contagiosa

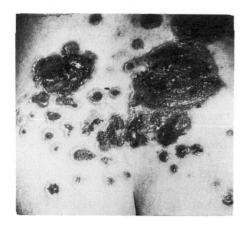

Impetigo contagiosa is an infectious superficial infection usually due, in temperate climates, to the staphylococcus or to mixed invasion by streptococci and staphylococci. In infants it can cause severe illness but in adults it is usually trivial. It often develops as a complication of a skin condition, especially eczema, but also commonly accompanies pediculosis or scabies. In the common variety superficial thin-roofed lakes of pus form on the face, hands, or knees and evolve rapidly into raw oozing areas which dry, leaving golden crusts. In the bullous variety large thick-walled blisters appear. The contents are initially clear but later purulent. The crusts should be removed gently by soaking with saline solution. The raw areas are then treated with a thin smear of 3% chlortetracycline ointment applied four times daily, and an oral antibiotic is given. The child should stay at home until the eruption has cleared.

Seborrhoeic dermatitis

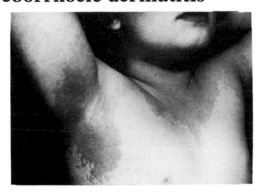

Seborrhoeic eczema is so called because it may occur in sites of increased sebaceous activity, the face, neck, chest, and back. Seborrhoea, however, or an abnormality of the sebaceous glands is not considered a feature of the condition. It occurs commonly in the first three months of life as an erythematous scaly eruption on the scalp and face, but any of the body folds may be affected, including the neck, axillae, and groin. There is no itching but secondary infection is common, particularly with *Candida*. In some children atopic eczema may follow seborrhoeic dermatitis, but the latter is not thought to be due to atopy.

Pityriasis alba

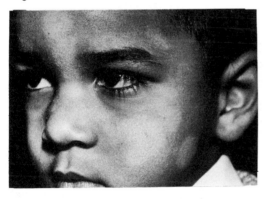

Pityriasis alba is a chronic eczema, which occurs predominantly in children as rounded or oval hypopigmented mildly scaly patches usually on the face but occasionally on the upper arms and back. It may be associated with atopic eczema or may occur alone. The patches are often multiple, and initial erythema is followed by hypopigmentation, which prompts the parents to seek advice. The eruption is self-limiting but may last two or three years. The scaling may be reduced by a bland cream and any inflammation treated with a weak topical steroid.

Napkin dermatitis (contact irritant type)

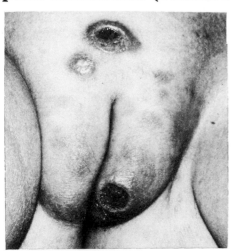

Neonatal skin is thinner than adult skin, has less eccrine and sebaceous gland secretions, and shows a depressed reactivity to contact allergens. It is more susceptible to external irritants and bacterial infection, and these combine with other factors to produce a contact dermatitis.

Prolonged contact with urine or faeces, maceration of skin induced by wet napkins and waterproof pants, and secondary infection with *Candida albicans* lead to an irritant dermatitis. Urea-splitting bacteria which release ammonia are encouraged by the warm, wet environment produced by impervious clothing. The dermatitis appears as a confluent erythema at sites closest to the napkin, usually with sparing of the folds, and readily becomes secondarily infected, producing pustules and erosions. In boys inflammation of the urinary meatus often occurs and may cause dysuria and urinary retention.

Napkin dermatitis is managed by keeping the area clean and dry and avoiding occlusive dressings. Plastic or rubber pants should not be used except for important occasions. Disposable napkins are

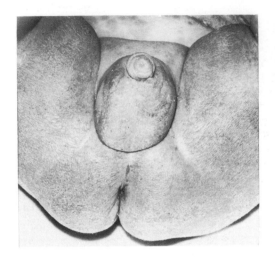

preferable to those which require plastic overpants, though some disposable napkins also have an outer plastic lining. Towelling napkins are best if thoroughly washed, rinsed and sterilised. A mild detergent is advisable and the rinse cycle of a washing machine needs to be completed twice. The napkins can be sterilised by soaking them in a chlorinated isocyanurate solution. Napkins must be changed often. Regular compresses of saline solution (one level teaspoonful of salt in a pint of water) can be applied if the dermatitis is acute and exudative, or the affected area can be exposed for two or three days. In the past ointments have been avoided for acute weeping dermatoses but they are as effective as creams when used in similar concentrations. A 1% hydrocortisone preparation is used three or four times daily for a week, but a more potent steroid such as triamcinolone may be necessary for severe dermatitis. Strong fluorinated steroids should be used only a week. Secondary bacterial infection is treated with both topical and oral antibiotics. Similarly monilial infection is treated by topical nystatin, and oral nystatin is also given to clear the intestinal reservoir of yeast. When the skin has recovered a barrier preparation such as zinc and castor oil ointment is applied with each nappy change to prevent recurrence.

"Lick eczema"

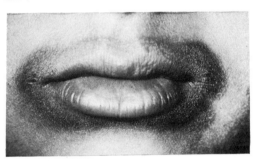

The site of a contact irritant dermatitis varies according to the cause. A reaction to a bubble bath, antiseptic agent, or tar sulphur soap may cause a widespread eruption, although the rash is often most prominent on the cheeks, neck, external surfaces of the limbs, and the buttocks. Lip licking or thumb sucking often causes a reaction due to saliva. The child and parents do not recognise the cause and notice a spreading irritating perioral eruption with fissuring. A mild steroid for a few days and then liberal applications of petroleum jelly help to clear the eruption. The eruption disappears when the child is persuaded to stop the habit.

Warts

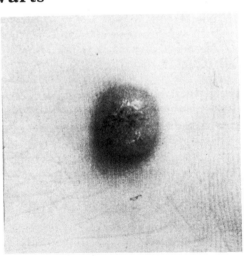

Human warts are caused by a papovavirus, to which children aged 6 to 12 years are particularly prone; 65% resolve within two years of their onset. Warts may occur anywhere on the body though most occur on the hands and feet. The verrucous mass will often show multiple thrombosed capillary loops which resemble black dots. Warts are destroyed by physical or chemical methods. The adage that the best way to manage warts is to let them manage themselves still seems appropriate. When treatment is necessary simple measures such as covering the lesion with a waterproof adhesive bandage changed daily should be tried initially. The next measure is to pare the surface of the wart with an emery board or pumice stone and apply a paint of 10–20% podophyllin in tincture of benzoic compound daily for two to six weeks. A little petroleum jelly smeared on the normal skin around the wart will protect it from any irritant effect. If these methods fail the wart may be frozen with liquid nitrogen as it avoids the need for local anaesthetic and does not produce the painful scar that often results from diathermy cautery or excision.

Molluscum contagiosum

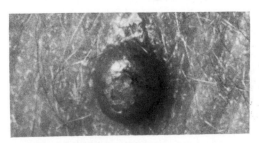

Molluscum contagiosum is caused by a pox virus and can spread rapidly. Multiple lesions are common in young children between the ages of 2 and 5 years and tend to occur especially on the face and trunk. The typical lesion is a dome-shaped flesh-coloured umbilicated papule which releases a cheesy white material when pierced and expressed. Molluscum contagiosum can resolve spontaneously. The lesions may be readily destroyed by piercing with a sharpened orange stick dipped in 10% podophyllin in industrial methylated spirit. Other equally effecive measures include gentle curettage and cryotherapy.

Pediculosis capitis

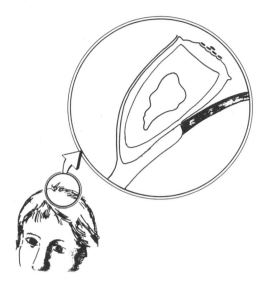

The eggshaped capsules (nits) and lice of pediculosis capitis infect the hair of the head and eyelashes and there may be secondary impetigo of the scalp.

There are several effective treatments. Gammabenzene hexachloride 1% in a shampoo base (Quellada PC Application) is applied to wet hair and rubbed in vigorously to produce a generous lather. The application is left on for four or five minutes and the hair then rinsed thoroughly. While the hair is still wet it is combed with a fine-toothed metal comb to remove dead lice and nits. One application is usually enough. Malathion, an organophosphorus compound, also available as a 1% cream shampoo, is less irritant to the skin than gammabenzene hydrochloride, and has a marked residual action on the hair, which is a further advantage. It is effective against certain strains of "superlice" resistant to other conventional therapy. Malathion in lotion form is inflammable and after its use the hair should be allowed to dry naturally. Artificial heat, e.g. electric hair dryers, should be avoided. As with other shampoos, it should not be allowed to touch the eyes or other mucous surfaces. Carbaryl lotion 0·5% is also effective against head lice. Children should be persuaded to avoid sharing each other's hats, caps, brushes, or combs and encouraged to have their hair washed frequently.

Scabies

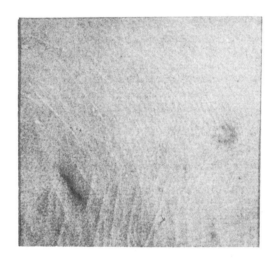

Scabies is caused by the ubiquitous mite *Sarcoptes scabiei* and the typical eruption consists of pruritic papules, vesicles, and burrows. The papules result from invasion of the larval stages of the parasite, the vesicles from host sensitisation, and the burrow marks the site of the adult female mite where it has dug into the horny layer of the epidermis. In adults and older children the eruption tends to favour the fingerwebs, flexor aspects of the wrists, axillae, and the genitalia. In infants and young children the distribution may include the palms and soles, the head, face, and neck, and burrows may be absent. Furthermore, bullae, which are uncommon in the adult, may occur in children.

Treatment consists of two topical applications of 1% gammabenzene hexachloride to all areas of the body, except the face and neck, with 24 hours between applications. All people occupying the same accommodation and other close contacts should be treated even if they do not show overt evidence of scabies. At the end of treatment intimate articles of clothing (underwear, pyjamas, sheets, and pillowcase) should be laundered and ironed. Even after adequate treatment pruritus may persist but this usually responds to 10% crotamiton cream used for a week or two. If this appears unsuccessful reinfection or an alternative cause should be considered.

Fungal infection

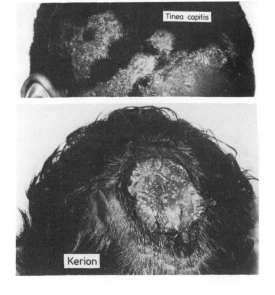

Tinea capitis

Kerion

Trichophyton tonsurans causes a diffuse hair loss with broken hairs. *Microsporum canis* or *Trichophyton mentagrophytes* may cause an acutely inflamed pustular mass containing few hairs—kerion. For confirmation of a fungal lesion of the skin, scales are obtained from the border of a lesion. Hairs infected with a microsporum species will fluoresce green when examined under a Wood's (long-wave UVL) lamp. In infections of the hair and nails a systemic antifungal agent, griseofulvin, is the treatment of choice, whereas for skin infections alone a topical antifungal agent is usually adequate. In the latter group the imidazole derivatives, clotrimazole and miconazole, have superseded the well-tried though cosmetically less acceptable benzoic acid compound (Whitfield's ointment) and Castellani's paint.

FEBRILE CONVULSIONS

Most of the fits which occur between the ages of 1 and 5 years are simple febrile convulsions and have an excellent prognosis. If there is no fever the possibility of epilepsy should be considered (see next chapter).

Often fever is recognised only when a convulsion has already occurred. An abrupt rise in temperature rather than a high level is important. There may be a frightened cry followed by abrupt loss of consciousness with muscular rigidity, which form the tonic stage. Cessation of respiratory movements and incontinence of urine and faeces may occur during this stage, which usually lasts up to half a minute. The clonic stage which follows consists of repetitive movements of the limbs or face. By arbitrary definition, in simple febrile convulsions the fit lasts less than 15 minutes, there are no focal features, and the child is aged between 1 and 5 years and has been developing normally.

Rigors may occur in any acute febrile illness, but there is no loss of consciousness.

Simple febrile convulsions

All the following:

   <15 minutes

   No focal features

   1–5 years

   Normal development

Emergency treatment

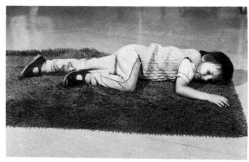

If the child has fever all his clothes should be removed and he should be covered with a sheet only. This applies whether the child is at home or in the accident and emergency department. If his temperature does not fall within a few minutes he can be sponged with cool water, a wet sheet can be applied to his trunk or he can be placed in a *shallow* bath of *cool, not* cold, water. He should be nursed on his side or prone with his head to one side because vomiting with aspiration is a constant hazard. It may be dangerous to take an ill febrile child into his parents' warm bed.

If convulsions are still occurring or start again paraldehyde with hyaluronidase should be given intramuscularly. A glass syringe is ideal, but if only a plastic syringe is available the paraldehyde should be injected within two minutes of filling the syringe. The dose of paraldehyde is 0·2 ml/kg; 1 ml of sterile water is added to an ampoule of hyaluronidase, and 0·1 ml of this solution is aspirated into the syringe containing the measured amount of paraldehyde and shaken well just before injection. If the dose of paraldehyde is over 2 ml it should be divided and given into two sites. The time the paraldehyde is given should be noted in writing.

If at home the child should then be transferred to hospital. If the convulsions do not stop within 10 minutes of giving paraldehyde the duty anaesthetist should be present while another drug is given intravenously. Diazepam (0·3 mg/kg) or a short-acting barbiturate must be given slowly over several minutes. Diazepam is an extremely effective anticonvulsant but the standard preparation cannot be diluted and it is difficult to measure accurately the small dose needed in infants. The use of a 1 ml tuberculin syringe allows small doses to be given slowly. If the dose is too large or is given too quickly, particularly if the patient has previously received an anticonvulsant,

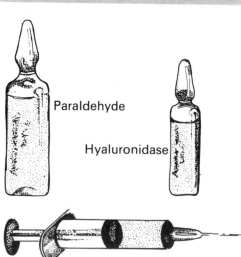

Paraldehyde

Hyaluronidase

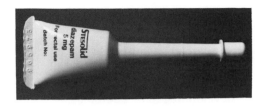

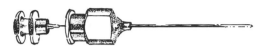

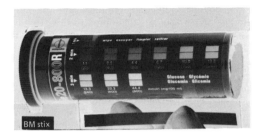

BM stix

there is a risk of respiratory arrest. A special preparation of diazepam for intravenous use (Diazemuls) can be diluted with glucose solution and can be measured more accurately. Early transfer to the intensive care unit should be considered if a second dose of anticonvulsant is needed.

Rectal diazepam (0·5 mg/kg) is a safe alternative to paraldehyde or intravenous diazepam and produces an effective blood concentration within 10 minutes. The most convenient preparation resembles a toothpaste tube (Stesolid). The alternative is to use the standard intravenous preparation with disposable syringes and short pieces of plastic tubing. The closed end of the sheath of a disposable needle can be cut off to provide a substitute for the plastic tubing. Parents should be taught how to give the chosen preparation.

All children who have had a first febrile convulsion should be admitted for lumbar puncture to exclude meningitis and to educate the parents, as many fear that their child is dying during the fit. Physical examination at this stage usually does not show a cause for the fever but a specimen of urine should be examined in the laboratory to exclude infection, and a blood culture and BM stix test should be performed. Most of these children have a generalised viral infection with viraemia. A febrile convulsion may occur in roseola at the onset and three days later the rash appears. Occasionally acute otitis media is present, in which case an antibiotic is indicated, but most children with febrile convulsions do not need an antibiotic.

Prognosis and long-term management

Febrile convulsions

Your child has had a febrile convulsion. This means that he (or she) had a fit because he had a high temperature. It is very common for this to happen (one child in 30 has one between the ages of 9 months and 5 years). The fit was very frightening for you but will not have harmed your child.

The following is general advice on how to handle him in future.

TEMPERATURE CONTROL

If he starts to develop a temperature:
1. Take off his clothes.
2. Give him regular paracetamol in the doses shown:
    Less than 1 year   1 × 5-ml spoonful every 6 hours
    Over 1 year   2 × 5-ml spoonfuls every 6 hours
3. To bring his temperature down it may be necessary to sponge him with tepid water for 5 minutes or place him in a *shallow* bath of cool, *not* cold, water.

REGULAR MEDICINE

Some children are more likely to have further fits than others and for them we recommend regular medicine to prevent this. The medicine has to be given every day until the child is about 3½ years, when it can possibly be stopped. Not every child needs regular medicine and a doctor will tell you if your child needs it. Each child on regular medicine has a blood test about 3 weeks after he starts it to check that the dose is right for him.

OTHER FITS

If your child does have another fit, don't worry! Lie him down where he cannot hurt himself, with his head face down, so that if he is actually sick it will not go into his lungs and his tongue will drop forward.

THEN—EITHER (a) Give rectal diazepam, OR
                  (b) Take him to your doctor, OR
                  (c) Call your doctor if he is likely to come quickly, OR
                  (d) Go to an accident and emergency department (in an emergency you can call an ambulance).

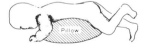

THE POSITION YOUR CHILD SHOULD BE PLACED IN IF HE HAS ANOTHER FIT.

Remember to keep all medicines out of the reach of children.

Febrile convulsions occur in about 3% of preschool children. Of the children with febrile convulsions, about a third will have further attacks, but fewer than 3% have convulsions after the age of 5 years. If they think he has fever, the parents are advised to cool the child by taking off his clothes and giving him paracetamol. A simple leaflet on the management of convulsions should be given to the parents and they should be shown how to give rectal diazepam.

A very large study showed that no patient with a simple febrile convulsion had a subsequent serious neurological disorder or intellectual impairment. Two-thirds of children with convulsions and fever have simple febrile convulsions, and no prophylactic drugs are indicated for them after the first attack. About 30% of children with febrile convulsions had a second episode and 10% had multiple episodes in this study. Prophylactic anticonvulsants should be considered for children who have had more than two fits and given until they reach the age of 3½ years. Continuous phenobarbitone (5 mg/kg) given only at bedtime is effective in reducing the incidence of recurrence but it produces irritability in some children and in these cases sodium valproate (20–30 mg/kg divided into two doses) can be substituted. The object is prevention of a recurrence of the harrowing experience of a convulsion for the parents as the long-term prognosis for the child is excellent with or without prophylactic drugs. Sodium valproate is not the first line drug as it is associated very rarely with hepatitis or pancreatitis. Phenytoin has no value in the prevention of febrile convulsions.

Febrile convulsions

Complex febrile convulsions

One or more of:
- >15 minutes
- Focal
- Repeated on the same day
- <1 year or >5 years
- Development or neurological abnormalities

Children who have had one "complex" convulsion should receive phenobarbitone or sodium valproate for two years after the last episode. "Complex" convulsions last over 15 minutes or are focal at the beginning or during the fit. Children with convulsions and with previous developmental or neurological abnormalities or a first degree relative with epilepsy should receive phenobarbitone or sodium valproate for at least two years.

Anticonvulsant blood values should be checked three weeks after the first dose and then every six months. Treatment should be withdrawn gradually over a few months.

EPILEPSY

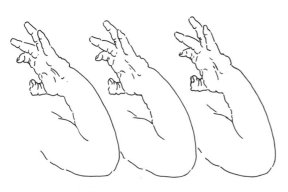

Recurrent attacks with similar features are essential for the diagnosis of epilepsy. The attacks may cause changes of consciousness or mood or produce abnormal sensory, motor, or visceral symptoms or signs. These changes are caused by recurring excessive neuronal discharges in the brain, although the electroencephalogram (EEG) may be normal. Investigations are no substitute for a history taken carefully from a witness. Documented absence of fever is essential to exclude the more common problem of febrile convulsions (see previous chapter). The incidence of epilepsy is about 6 in 1000 schoolchildren compared with the incidence of children with febrile convulsions, which is about 30 per 1000 preschool children. A single seizure may need investigation but should not be called epilepsy and specific treatment is usually not indicated.

Disability depends partly on the frequency and severity of the fits but also on the presence or absence of developmental delay, cerebral palsy or defects in the special senses which would suggest brain damage. The word "damage" will be used in this chapter, but for discussion with parents "abnormality" is preferred. Most children with epilepsy attend normal schools, rarely have fits and have no disability apart from the fits.

Epileptic fits can be divided into generalised or partial seizures. Generalised seizures include grand and petit mal and myoclonic fits. Partial seizures include focal and temporal lobe fits.

Check

developmental level

motor function

hearing

sight (including squint)

skin (tuberose sclerosis)

Grand mal

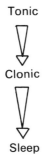

Tonic

Clonic

Sleep

Sodium valproate

Carbamazepine

Phenytoin

About 80% of children with epilepsy have grand mal (tonic–clonic) seizures. The child may appear irritable or show other unusual behaviour for a few minutes or even for hours before an attack. Sudden loss of consciousness occurs during the tonic phase, which lasts 20–30 seconds and is accompanied by temporary cessation of respiratory movements and central cyanosis. The clonic phase follows and there are jerking movement of limbs and face. The movements gradually stop and the child may sleep for a few minutes before waking, confused and irritable. The best prognosis occurs in older children and those who respond promptly to anticonvulsants. When epilepsy is secondary to brain damage the prognosis may be less good. Sodium valproate and phenytoin are the commonly used drugs. Carbamazepine has special value in children with brain damage. Anticonvulsants are given until two to four years have passed with no symptoms and then discontinued gradually over several months.

Epilepsy

Petit mal

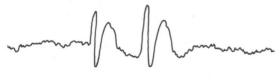

In petit mal episodes of altered consciousness lasting 10–15 seconds occur spontaneously and can be precipitated by hyperventilation. Petit mal is rarely associated with mental retardation or brain damage. There is a typical EEG appearance, and the frequent attacks respond promptly to ethosuximide or to sodium valproate introduced slowly. Treatment is continued for two years after the fits have been controlled.

Myoclonic epilepsy

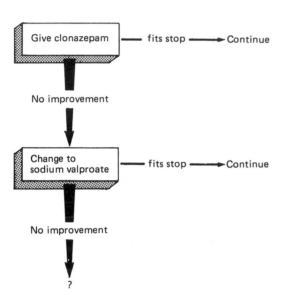

Myoclonic epilepsy is caused by different brain insults; heredity may be implicated. Many of these children have developmental delay and some evidence of brain abnormality before the fits begin. The child may have a variety of seizures including (a) symmetrical synchronous flexion movements (myoclonic); (b) brief loss of consciousness; and (c) sudden head-dropping attacks (atonic–akinetic). Infantile spasms are a form of myoclonic epilepsy which starts before the age of 1 year, has a characteristic EEG, and is treated with a course of ACTH or prednisolone.

Perinatal asphyxia or acquired brain damage from any cause may have been present. Many of the children have mental retardation but the degree is variable. The EEG may remain normal long after the onset of the symptoms. Myoclonic epilepsy must be distinguished from petit mal epilepsy as treatment and prognosis are different.

Myoclonic seizures are often difficult to control with drugs. Clonazepam is introduced gradually until the attacks cease or drowsiness occurs. Sodium valproate is usually the next drug used. As a last resort it may be necessary to use a combination of various drugs or a ketogenic diet.

Partial seizures

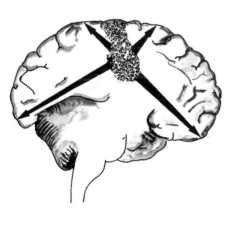

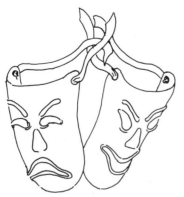

Partial seizures originate in specific areas of the brain and the symptoms depend on the site of the epileptic focus. Perinatal asphyxia or prolonged "complex" febrile convulsions are the main cause; a progressive space-occupying lesion is an extremely rare cause of this clinical picture. The commonest variety of partial epilepsy in childhood is benign focal epilepsy of childhood where the focus is in the Rolandic area. It usually starts between the ages of 7 and 10 years and attacks begin especially during sleep. Often they become generalised so that any generalised nocturnal convulsions may be due to this conditon, which has a good prognosis. Consciousness is often retained but the child does not speak or swallow during the attack. There may be jerking of one side of the face with salivation, gurgling noises, and peculiar sensations affecting the tongue. Carbamazepine is extremely effective and most of the children are completely free of fits and then need no drugs shortly after puberty. Phenytoin is given with carbamazepine if the fits continue despite the single drug treatment.

In contrast, the great variety of bizarre symptoms produced by fits originating in the temporal lobe makes diagnosis difficult and attacks may be intractable despite anticonvulsants. There may be short episodes of emotional disturbance with the sudden onset of fear or rage, hallucinations of sight, sound, or smell or visceral symptoms such as epigastric discomfort. A generalised tonic–clonic seizure may follow in some children. Carbamazepine is effective in about half the patients and is introduced slowly over several weeks to avoid drowsiness and ataxia. Phenytoin is the next drug to be tried. Rarely surgical removal of the temporal lobe has been performed and is effective in about 50% of children when medical treatment has failed to control the fits. The best surgical results occur when histology shows mesial temporal sclerosis, which follows prolonged "complex" febrile convulsions.

Differential diagnosis

Febrile convulsions

Breath-holding attacks

Syncope

Acute labyrinthitis

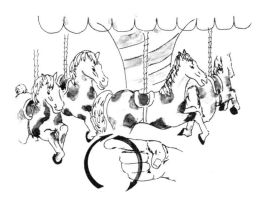

Breath-holding attacks—Convulsions need to be differentiated from breath-holding attacks, which usually begin at 9 to 18 months. Immediately after a frustrating or painful experience the child cries vigorously and then suddenly holds his breath, becomes cyanosed or pale, and in the most severe cases loses consciousness. Rarely his limbs become rigid, and there may be a few clonic movements lasting a few seconds. He takes a deep breath and regains consciousness immediately. The attacks diminish with age and there is no specific treatment. Mothers may be helped to manage these extremely frightening episodes by being told that the child will not die and that they should handle each attack consistently by putting the child down on his side.

Syncope or a faint may occur at any age but is more usual in older children. While in the upright position the child appears very pale, becomes unsteady, and falls to the ground. There may be a precipitating factor such as standing in one position for a long time or being in a closed, hot room. Rarely there may be a few clonic movements of the limbs but never a generalised convulsion and within a few minutes the child is perfectly normal again. He may say that he felt dizzy or unsteady at the beginning of the attack. Isolated episodes with obvious precipitating factors require no treatment.

Acute labyrinthitis is another cause of episodes of dizziness. The child is frightened and may fall or vomit but does not lose consciousness. If he is asked to draw his sensation in the air with his finger he will describe a circular movement which suggests vertigo. This is due to a viral infection affecting the balance mechanism of the inner ear which usually resolves within a few weeks, although attacks occasionally persist for longer.

Investigations

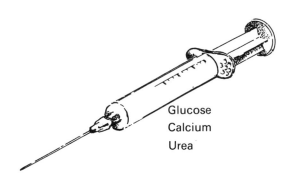

Glucose
Calcium
Urea

Investigations should be performed as outpatient procedures, keeping them to the minimum necessary for making a firm diagnosis and for excluding treatable causes. The specific tests will depend on the diagnosis made after taking the history and examining fasting plasma glucose, calcium, and urea concentrations. A BM stix test should be performed during a fit and if abnormal, blood is taken for a blood glucose estimation.

Radiology of the skull may show abnormal calcification. The EEG should not be used to determine whether a child has epilepsy; this is a clinical decision. But the EEG may provide guidance on the type of epilepsy so that appropriate drugs are given, or it may show a unilateral lesion indicating the need for a brain scan by computerised axial tomography. Other indications for brain scan in children with fits are controversial, but an abnormality can be shown in a higher proportion of children with additional factors such as developmental delay or partial seizures. The EEG does not show whether the epilepsy is improving or whether it is safe to stop treatment.

General management

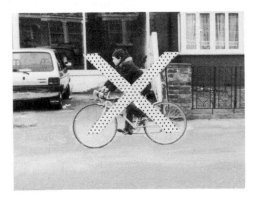

Regular measurements of blood or salivary anticonvulsant levels may help to prevent side effects and confirm compliance but the dose must be determined mainly by the presence or absence of fits. The majority of children need only two doses of anticonvulsant each day and a single drug is the ideal.

An adult must be present constantly at bath-time and it is safer if the water is shallow (5–7·5 cm). Children with epilepsy should not ride a bicycle in the open road or swim unless there is an adult with them in the water. They should not climb ropes or high bars in a gymnasium. They can carry out all other activities. The schoolteacher needs to know the child's diagnosis and be aware that most children with epilepsy have normal intelligence and should be expected to perform as well as their peers.

Epilepsy

```
2+3=6
5−1=3

1   Anticonvulsant blood level ↑
2   Fits++
3   Intelligence ↓
```

Learning difficulties may be due to the effects of anticonvulsants, inattention caused by unrecognised fits or underlying brain damage. Epilepsy is a family problem which can modify the lives of all members and the parents will be worried about the child's prospects for future employment, driving a car, and marriage. They may believe, wrongly, that epilepsy is always associated with mental retardation. The doctor should tell the parents that the fits are *not* due to a tumour, that the child will *not* die in an attack, and that a short fit does *not* injure the brain.

RECURRENT HEADACHE

Any acute illness with pyrexia may cause headache, but if there is drowsiness, vomiting, photophobia, neck stiffness, or purpura an emergency lumbar puncture needs to be considered to exclude meningitis. Recurrent headaches are due to migraine, emotional tension, muscle contraction, or intracranial pathology. Emotional factors may precipitate attacks of migraine. Muscle contraction headaches occur if there is repeated clenching or grinding of the teeth. Detailed physical examination is essential on the first visit, and reassessment is needed during the first six months after the onset of headaches to exclude a cerebral tumour which did not produce localising symptoms or signs initially. The blood pressure should be measured and the fundi examined in every child with headache. Migraine occurs in about 4% of children, and tension headaches probably have about the same incidence.

- Migraine
- Emotional tension
- Muscle contraction
- Intracranial pathology

Migraine

	Mon	Tue	Wed	Thur	Fri	Sat	Sun	Mon	Tue	W
08.00										
10.00	//							//		
12.00	//					//		//		
14.00	//					//		//		
16.00	//							//		
18.00										

//// Headache

The pain of migraine is usually accompanied by nausea or vomiting and is relieved by sleep. There is often intolerance to light or noise and there may be marked pallor. The pain lasts for hours and there is complete freedom from pain between attacks. In about 20% of the patients there is a hemicranial distribution of the pain, and in about another 20% there is vertigo or light-headedness. Only about 5% of children with migraine have a visual aura. Migraine can occur at any age, but it is rare under the age of 5 years.

Ninety per cent of children with migraine have parents or siblings with this condition, so the absence of a family history throws some doubt on the diagnosis. As 50% of all children have a family history of migraine the *presence* of this history is not helpful in diagnosis. Although they may have been called migraine, the details of the relatives' headaches may show that they have the features of emotional tension headaches.

Psychological stress is the commonest trigger factor of attacks, and school is often implicated. The child may have difficulty in keeping up with his peers or may fear impending examinations. Children are often seen by a doctor for the first time at the beginning of the new school year in September, but in other families the mother may cope until March or April. Some of these children are progressing well at school but pursue a very hectic life afterwards. The importance of specific foods is controversial but a mother may have observed that a particular food such as chocolate or cheese may consistently precipitate symptoms. This occurs in about 10% of children. Provided only one type of food is implicated, it can be excluded from the diet. Any more extensive alterations should be supervised by a paediatric dietitian. A head injury or acute upper respiratory tract infection may precipitate a series of attacks, but the importance of acute sinusitis either as a trigger factor in migraine or as a specific cause of recurrent headache has probably been exaggerated. Physical activity to exhaustion, mild hypoglycaemia due to missing a meal, excessive exposure to sun, or a lack of sleep may precipitate attacks in susceptible children.

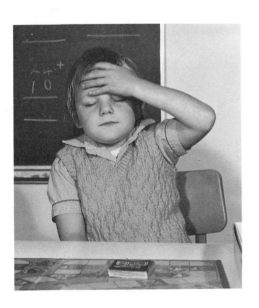

Recurrent headache

Management

There are no abnormal signs on examination and no investigations are indicated when the diagnosis is clear clinically. The diagnosis is explained to the whole family, including the child, and it is pointed out that most children have exacerbations of six months' duration within a 2–4 year period of school-related exacerbations followed by a remission which may last between nine years and indefinitely. Avoidance of trigger factors may need exploration with the help of a school report and sometimes assessment by a psychologist. If the symptoms have been present for less than six months a further physical examination will be needed until enough time has elapsed to exclude an intracranial lesion. Although this possibility needs to be considered, it need not be transmitted to the parents, but many parents will be worried about the possibility of a tumour and the value of a normal examination can be emphasised.

Treatment of an acute attack is more likely to be effective if it is given early. A supply of an antiemetic (for example, metoclopramide) and paracetamol should be kept at school as well as at home. If this is not effective the child should be allowed to lie down in a darkened room for half an hour. If there are several attacks each week regular continuous prophylactic treatment with propranolol may be recommended for six months by a paediatrician. Behaviour modification techniques have been successful where parents are motivated and staff with the necessary skills are available.

Emotional tension

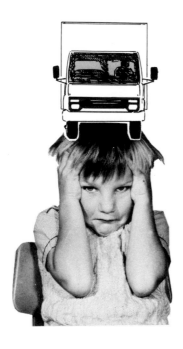

The headache is often present every day, usually starting in the afternoon and continuing to the evening. It is described as an ache, tightness, or pressure affecting any part of the head. It is commonly frontal but may be felt in the temporal or occipital regions. Poor school attendance is common, with absence from school for weeks at a time. Evidence of environmental factors causing anxiety at school and at home should be sought, and there may be additional physical symptoms such as pain in the abdomen or limbs which complete the picture. There may be overt symptoms of psychiatric disturbance such as depression, disruptive behaviour in group activities, or destruction of property.

Management

The absence of physical signs confirms the diagnosis and helps the family to accept it. Specific investigations are seldom required, but a further assessment is needed to allow the parents to consider any further relevant factors, to discuss the school report with them, to plan further management, and to confirm the absence of abnormal physical signs if the history is short. Simple changes in the child's routine or environment or, occasionally, referral to a child psychiatrist, may be needed.

Intracranial lesions

Most intracranial lesions are cerebral tumours or vascular malformations, but a few are subdural haemorrhages or intracranial abscesses. These lesions do not produce a specific clinical picture, but there are some pointers which make the diagnosis more likely.

Abnormal physical signs are present in the majority of children with intracranial lesions either when they are first seen or within four months of the onset of symptoms. About half of the children have papilloedema, and other common signs are disturbances in gait or hemiparesis. Headache which wakes the child at night, is present on waking in the morning, or is aggravated by coughing suggests an intracranial lesion.

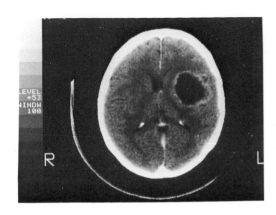

The following are indications for referral to a paediatrician or paediatric neurologist, who will usually arrange computed tomography of the brain as the first investigation.

(1) Abnormal neurological signs during or after headache.
(2) Fits with headache.
(3) Nocturnal or early morning headache, especially if the history is shorter than six months or if the headaches are increasing in frequency or severity.
(4) Recent school failure, change in behaviour—especially apathy or irritability—or failure to grow in height.
(5) Change in quality or distribution of headache.
(6) Extremely severe incapacitating headaches.
(7) Age less than 5 years.

POISONING

Accidental swallowing of drugs and household fluids is common among children, especially between the ages of 2 and 3 years. Most of them take trivial amounts of drugs, but every child must be assessed carefully to ensure that effective treatment is given when a potentially fatal dose has been swallowed. A health visitor's report on the family may be helpful as the event may indicate a chaotic household or a non-accidental injury. Child-resistant containers have reduced the incidence of poisoning by tablets.

The name of the drug may be on the bottle, or the tablets may be identifiable from charts. The prescriber, hospital pharmacist, or the pharmacist who dispensed the tablets may be able to help. The time the drug was taken should be written in the clinical notes and whether any symptoms such as vomiting have occurred. The maximum amount of drug that could have been taken should be estimated. The original number of tablets in the bottle may be known. Usually the dispensing pharmacist knows the original number of tablets dispensed.

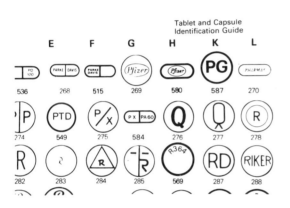

Tablet and Capsule Identification Guide

Non poisons

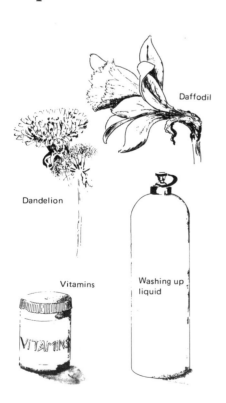

Daffodil

Dandelion

Vitamins

Washing up liquid

Accidental ingestion of a substance known to be non-poisonous can be dealt with by reassurance alone.

Antibiotics, vitamins, simple antacids, and oral contraceptives are not toxic. Homeopathic preparations are non-toxic but must be distinguished from herbal preparations, which may contain enough active substances to cause symptoms.

Mild diarrhoea or vomiting may occur after the ingestion of plants, but most are non-toxic. Berries that are non-toxic include those of berberis, Chinese lantern, cotoneaster, hawthorn, mahonia, mountain ash (rowan), pyracantha, skimmia, and japonica. Most flowers are non-toxic—for example, antirrhinum, daffodil, bluebell, daisy, dandelion, fuschia, geranium, rose, violet, stock.

Bathsoap, bubble bath, carpet cleaner, scouring powders, and dishwashing liquid are not toxic; however, dishwashing *powders* are highly alkaline. Innocuous water-based paints must be distinguished from oil-based paints in which the hydrocarbon solvents may be dangerous. Similarly, water-based glues are innocuous.

Nail varnish and nail varnish remover contain toxic solvents and perfumes contain alcohol, but the small amounts ingested are rarely enough to cause harm.

Anticoagulant rat baits such as Warfarin are toxic only in massive or repeated doses, so a serious change in prothrombin time due to acute poisoning is very unusual. Many weedkillers and pesticides are relatively harmless in small amounts, but some can be toxic and it is important to find out the ingredients in each case.

Examination

Level of consciousness

Respiratory rate

Blood pressure

Initially, maintaining adequate ventilation and circulation is more important than making an exact diagnosis. The level of consciousness is the most important single sign (see section on barbiturates below). The frequency and depth of the respiratory movements are noted. Slow, shallow movements suggest impending respiratory arrest and the need for assisted ventilation. A low blood pressure indicates that cardiac arrest is imminent.

Particles of tablets may be present in the mouth or vomit. The odour of paraffin (kerosene) may be present in the breath. Caustic or acid substances may cause burns on the lips and tongue and in the mouth. Deep sighing respiratory movements or a raised respiratory rate suggests salicylate poisoning, while tachycardia and dilated pupils are found in atropine poisoning. Opiates cause constriction of the pupils.

General management

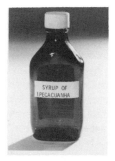

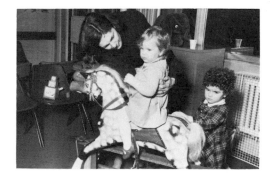

If the child is drowsy or unconscious a member of the paediatric unit should be called or the patient admitted to the intensive care unit. The following are contraindications to both induced vomiting and gastric lavage: (a) deterioration in the level of consciousness; (b) poisoning with paraffin, caustics, or acids.

If no contraindication is present the child should be given 15 ml of paediatric ipecacuanha emetic mixture followed by about 200 ml of water, which may be flavoured to taste. Paediatric ipecacuanha emetic mixture is a safe preparation. The child should walk around the room or be put on a rocking horse. If he does not vomit after about 20 minutes the same dose of ipecacuanha syrup and water is repeated. If emesis has been successful this should be noted in the clinical notes. Admission depends on the amount and the type of substance which has been taken (see below). In the few children who do not vomit after the second dose of ipecacuanha gastric lavage should be performed.

The poison may be known from the bottle or by identifying the tablets from charts. A specimen of vomit and of urine should be kept for possible analysis. Heparinised tubes should be used for collecting blood for salicylate estimation. The types of blood specimens required for estimating other poisons depend on the methods used in that laboratory.

Gastric lavage

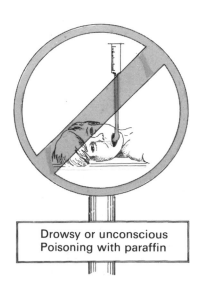

Drowsy or unconscious
Poisoning with paraffin

If the child is drowsy or unconscious gastric lavage should be postponed until an anaesthetist or paediatrician has ensured the security of the airway as there is a serious danger of aspiration into the lungs. The child should be wrapped in a blanket with his arms well secured and held firmly in the prone or left lateral position with his head lower than his trunk. The suction apparatus must be fitted with an adequate pharyngeal suction catheter, for example, FG 14, and must be shown to be working before the gastric tube is passed. The length of tube needed to reach the stomach is estimated by measuring the distance from the mouth to the ear lobe and from there to the lower end of the sternum. A tube of adequate bore, at least FG 24, is passed through the mouth into the stomach and the gastric contents are aspirated and a portion kept for later analysis.

Fifty ml of 1·4% sodium bicarbonate solution is allowed to pass into the stomach by gravity from the barrel of a 50-ml syringe. After a few minutes a similar volume is aspirated from the stomach by gravity or by using the 50-ml syringe. The procedure is repeated until about 500 ml has been used. The child is then admitted to the ward.

Poisoning

Salicylate poisoning

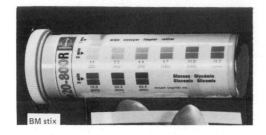

BM stix

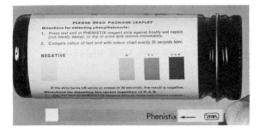

Phenistix

The incidence of aspirin poisoning has fallen since the introduction of child-proof containers. If aspirin has been given to treat an acute illness the toxic effects may be attributed to that illness. Infants may become more severely ill than older children even when the blood salicylate concentration is similar. Poisoning may result from the cumulative effect of frequent therapeutic doses. Vomiting and deep respiratory movements are early signs of salicylate poisoning and may mimic pneumonia, while drowsiness and coma are late features.

Methyl salicylate (oil of wintergreen) used as an embrocation in adults is dangerous, as only 4 ml may be fatal in infants. The child can usually tolerate a single acute ingestion of 100 mg of aspirin/kg body weight without serious effect and if there is no doubt that he has taken a smaller amount than this he need not be admitted to hospital. If the dose is uncertain the child must be admitted. Aspirin is one of the few drugs where there is benefit from delayed gastric lavage, even 12 to 24 hours after ingestion. When facilities are available measuring blood salicylate concentrations may be helpful in management. Blood concentration should be estimated six hours after ingestion and again several hours later to ensure that it is not continuing to rise. If the plasma salicylate concentration is over 300 mg/l (2·2 mmol/l) the child has moderate or severe poisoning.

A BM stix test should be carried out to detect hypoglycaemia or hyperglycaemia. Urine from a child who has taken salicylate turns Phenistix brownish red or purple. Absence of this colour change when the tablets were taken at least six hours earlier excludes salicylate poisoning. The urine of a child who is receiving desferrioxamine for iron poisoning also changes Phenistix to brownish red. Children with severe salicylate poisoning need intravenous fluids and partial correction of the severe metabolic acidosis.

Barbiturates

Grading of levels of consciousness
Fully conscious
Drowsy but responds to verbal stimulation
No response to verbal stimuli, localised response to painful stimuli
No response to verbal stimuli, generalised response to painful stimuli
No response to painful stimuli

Management after ingestion of barbiturates, benzodiazepines, and other sedative or hypnotic drugs is similar. As the smallest dose of barbiturates ingested is usually an adult dose the child must be admitted. The timing of the onset of symptoms depends on the type of barbiturate. Repeat estimations of the level of consciousness are essential for management and can be recorded as in the chart.

The child must be nursed prone or on his side to avoid aspirating vomit. Slow, shallow respiratory movements are signs of impending respiratory arrest. Hundred per cent oxygen can be given by mask or inflatable bag with mask, such as an Ambu bag. An anaesthetist should be called immediately, and intubation and mechanical ventilation may be needed. Debris should be removed from the mouth with gauze swabs or by suction. Hypotension is treated initially by giving intravenous fluids to restore the central venous pressure.

If the child is drowsy or unconscious an emetic or gastric lavage should be considered by a senior member of the paediatric unit. An anaesthetist should be present for either of these procedures if there is any drowsiness. If the level of consciousness is normal emesis is induced.

Estimations of blood barbiturate concentrations do not help management but may be useful if there is doubt about the diagnosis. Clinical features are the best guide.

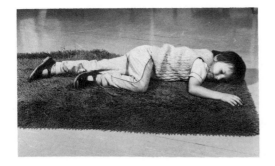

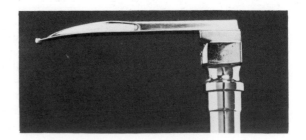

Paracetamol

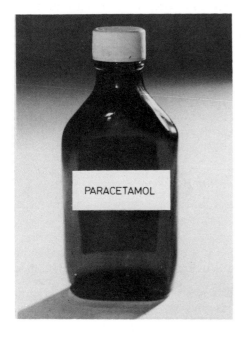

Serious toxicity occurs when more than about 150 mg/kg body weight of paracetamol has been taken. The initial features are nausea and pallor but there may be some improvement over the next 48 hours before the features of hepatic necrosis appear in severe poisoning. Necrosis is shown by jaundice, an enlarged tender liver, hypotension, and arrhythmias. Excitement and delirium may be followed by sudden coma, which is usually fatal. Hypothermia, hyperthermia, hypoglycaemia, or metabolic acidosis may occur.

Initial management is similar to that in barbiturate poisoning. Oral methionine or *N*-acetylcysteine (intravenous) given *within 10 hours* of the ingestion of paracetamol can reduce the incidence of liver necrosis in children with moderate or severe poisoning. If the child is vomiting or drowsy an intravenous preparation is preferable. As this treatment is only effective if given early, it is started if the history suggests that a large dose of paracetamol was taken. A blood paracetamol level is measured about four hours after ingestion as earlier samples are unreliable as a guide to treatment. This specific treatment should be continued if the plasma paracetamol concentration is above a line joining 200 mg/l at 4 hours and 70 mg/l 12 hours after ingestion. These high plasma concentrations are usually confined to older children who have attempted suicide. Intravenous bicarbonate may be needed to correct severe metabolic acidosis and intravenous glucose for hypoglycaemia.

Tricyclic drugs

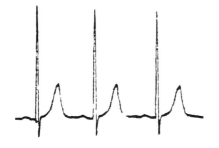

Amitriptyline and imipramine are widely used to treat depression in adults. An overdose of the paediatric syrup may be taken by a child being treated for enuresis. Drowsiness occurs within a few hours interrupted by periods of restlessness. Ataxia and tachycardia follow. If the child has taken more than 10 mg/kg body weight of amitriptyline or imipramine, convulsions, coma, and respiratory depression occur rapidly. Hypotension and cardiac arrhythmias may occur and the child should be observed with a cardiac monitor in the intensive care unit. Diazepam is effective in controlling convulsions.

Phenothiazines

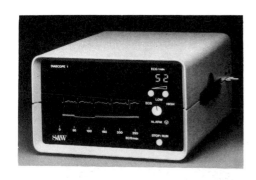

The phenothiazines include chlorpromazine, which is used as a sedative, piperazine, used to treat threadworms, and perphenazine, prescribed as an antiemetic.

Drowsiness is common and is managed as in barbiturate poisoning. The effects may resemble those of meningitis and there may be dyskinetic movements, including torticollis, facial grimacing, and abnormal eye movements. There may be symptoms similar to those seen in Parkinson's disease with muscular rigidity and tremor. Hypotension and hypothermia are common. The clinical features are similar to those of acute encephalitis or tetanus but there is no trismus.

Various cardiac arrhythmias may develop, and the electrocardiogram often shows prolongation of the Q-T interval and flattening of the T waves. The diagnosis may be confirmed by examining the urine for phenothiazine. General treatment is similar to that of barbiturate poisoning; cardiac arrhythmias are treated with an appropriate drug such as lignocaine or propranolol. Dyskinetic movements or convulsions can be treated with the chemical antagonist procyclidine (0·5–2 mg intravenously for under 2 year olds and 2–5 mg for 2 to 10 year olds; the ampoule should be diluted to 10 ml with isotonic saline solution). The dose should be repeated after 20 minutes if the symptoms have not been relieved.

Poisoning

Iron

Always admit

? Desferrioxamine

A toddler may take his mother's iron tablets prescribed for pregnancy. Swallowing a large number may be followed by necrosis of the gastrointestinal wall and rapid absorption of iron. During the first few hours after ingestion there may be vomiting, haematemesis and melaena, and severe abdominal pain accompanied by low blood pressure. After about 6 to 24 hours restlessness, convulsions, coma, and further haemorrhage may occur with metabolic acidosis and hepatic necrosis. *All* children who have ingested iron tablets should be admitted and kept in hospital for 48 hours because there may be a transient and deceptive improvement. A blood concentration of over 90 µmol/l (500 µg/100 ml) suggests serious poisoning, but low levels cannot be considered safe as there may be rapid deposition of iron in the liver.

Blood should be taken for urgent serum iron estimation and grouping and cross-matching of blood. Gastric lavage should be performed with desferrioxamine and treatment with intramuscular and intravenous desferrioxamine considered.

Alcohol

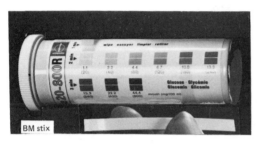

BM stix

Some children are particularly susceptible to the hypoglycaemic effects of alcohol, and any child who has taken even a small wine glass of ordinary wine should therefore be admitted to hospital for frequent feeds containing glucose or a continuous intravenous infusion of 10% glucose. The blood glucose concentration must be monitored by BM stix readings at least three hourly for the first 24 hours.

Belladonna alkaloids

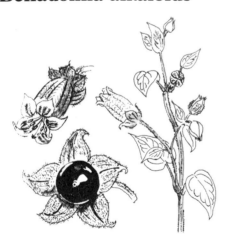

The belladonna alkaloids include atropine, hyoscine, and deadly nightshade. A child who has taken an overdose of any of these will have dilated pupils, a dry skin and mouth, fever, tachycardia, abdominal distention, excitement, and confusion. Admission for 48 hours is essential, though drug treatment is rarely necessary.

The commonest cause of an overdose of atropine is when the child takes too much Lomotil, which consists of diphenoxylate hydrochloride with atropine. With the addition of respiratory depression, the symptoms are the same as in atropine poisoning alone, except that the pupils are small. The diphenoxylate, which is an opioid, can be antagonised by naloxone; the dose of 0·2 mg IV may be repeated after about three minutes if there is no improvement. This dose is safe for children of all ages.

Paraffin or turpentine

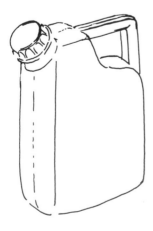

Although poisoning with paraffin is common, deaths, which are mainly due to respiratory complications, are rare. Turpentine is distilled from wood and differs chemically from paraffin but produces similar effects. Aspiration of paraffin into the lungs during ingestion or vomiting are the main dangers so emesis or gastric lavage should be avoided. There may be an increased respiratory rate, dyspnoea, and adventitious sounds, but extensive radiographic changes may be present with only slight symptoms. Radiological changes, which are usually bilateral, show patchy areas of consolidation in both lower lobes. Admission is always necessary as it may take 12 hours or more for the pulmonary features to appear.

Antihistamines

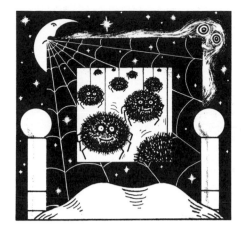

Some examples are chlorpheniramine, diphenhydramine, and promethazine. The clinical signs result from both excitation and depression of the central nervous system. Drowsiness and headache may be followed by fixed dilated pupils, incoordination, hallucinations, excitement, and convulsions. Other effects include hypotension, tachycardia, and occasionally cardiac arrhythmias, respiratory depression, or hyperpyrexia. The principles of treatment are similar to those of barbiturate poisoning. There is no specific antidote. Central nervous system excitation can be treated with diazepam.

For information and advice in cases of poisoning contact the following centres and ask for "poisons" information

National Poisons Information Service

Guy's Hospital	Ordinary enquiries	01-407 7600
London	Emergency enquiries	01-635 9191
Belfast	Royal Victoria Hospital	0232 40503
Cardiff	Cardiff Royal Infirmary	0222 569200
Dublin	Jervis Street Hospital	Dublin 745588
Edinburgh	Edinburgh Royal Infirmary	031-229 2477

Poisons information is also available from other centres:

Birmingham	Dudley Road Hospital	021-554 3801
Leeds	Leeds General Infirmary	0532 432799
Newcastle	Royal Victoria Infirmary	0632 325131

Examples of features suggesting a specific poison

Coma—Sedatives and anticonvulsants, salicylate alcohol, antihistamines.
Convulsion—Tricyclic antidepressants, amphetamines, antihistamines, alcohol.
Hallucinations—Belladonna group, amphetamines, antihistamines.
Involuntary movements—Phenothiazines, metoclopramide, antihistamines.
Small pupils—Opioids, diphenoxylate.
Large pupils—Belladonna, amphetamines, antihistamines, tricyclic antidepressants.
Tachycardia—Amphetamines, belladonna group.
Arrhythmias—Tricyclic antidepressants, phenothiazines.
Haematemesis—Caustic agents, iron.

ACCIDENTS

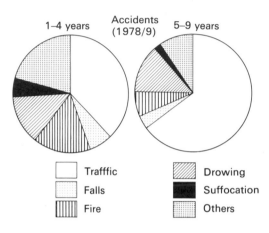

1–4 years   Accidents (1978/9)   5–9 years

- ☐ Trafffic
- ☐ Falls
- ☐ Fire
- ▨ Drowing
- ■ Suffocation
- ▨ Others

Accidents are the largest single cause of death between the ages of 1 and 15 years, causing more deaths than the two next commonest causes combined. Road accidents form the largest group followed by those in the home. Family doctors see as many patients with accidents as accident and emergency doctors, so a substantial proportion of children need medical attention for trauma every year. Non-accidental injury and poisoning will not be dealt with here.

The word "accident" implies that the event is not predictable or preventable. But prevention can be tackled by dividing the problem into factors concerning the child, the specific agent, and the circumstances. Since accidents in the home form a large proportion of accidents, it may be possible to prevent a future death by pointing out possible hazards for children during a home visit. Health visitors, who routinely visit homes with young children, also play an important part in suggesting how the home can be made more safe.

Road accidents

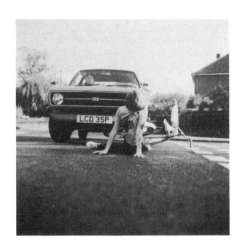

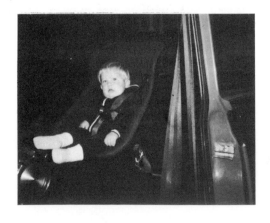

Traffic is the most complicated environment that a child can experience. Children are unable to anticipate all types of hazards in traffic and do not know how to adapt to them.

Nearly 80% of children aged 5 to 9 years who are killed or seriously injured in road accidents are pedestrians, compared with 28% of road accident casualties of all ages. Parents should be taught that young children cannot judge traffic properly and need to be accompanied in busy traffic. Many accidents are caused by children dashing out into the road when vision is obstructed. Studies have shown that children conform to guidelines on safe behaviour better than adults, but adults' behaviour is often far from ideal, and they might influence children to copy them. The risk of an accident while crossing the road decreases from 5 to 11 years, and the higher proportion of accidents in boys aged 5–7 than in girls may result from differences in behaviour, skills, and exposure during play.

One way of reducing bicycle accidents in children may be to make possession of a cycling proficiency certificate compulsory before a child is allowed to ride unaccompanied on a public road. Certainly children should be able to handle their bicycles properly, to look behind them, and to make signals before they are allowed on roads, and parents should ensure that the cycle is of the right size and properly maintained. Campaigns to improve adults' understanding of children's behaviour in traffic have been implemented in Sweden.

Children are injured less often in car accidents than adults and are safer in the rear seats than in the front. It is illegal for a child under 14 to sit unrestrained in the front of a car. An infant in a carry-cot placed transversely across the car can be protected by a restraint that attaches the carry-cot to the structure of the car and prevents the child from falling out of the cot during impact or when the car is inverted. When the child is old enough to sit up he can be carried in a properly designed and secured safety chair. Such a chair also allows small children to see out of the car windows. When the child outgrows this chair a child safety harness can be used.

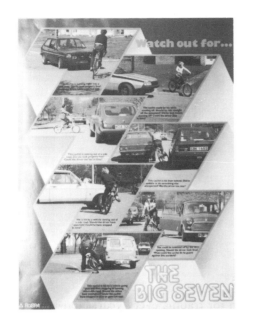

Pictorial teaching aids are widely used in schools to help increase children's awareness of road safety, but in many cases they are merely put up for children to see and it is important that children can understand them. Much research has been done into producing effective teaching material for use by teachers and children, but the value of this material cannot be determined for several years. This work has been sponsored by the Royal Society for the Prevention of Accidents (RoSPA), the Transport and Road Research Laboratory, the Child Accident Prevention Committee, as well as the Health Education Council.

Accidents in the home

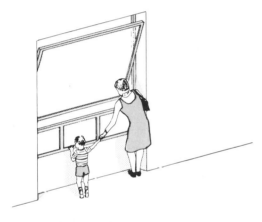

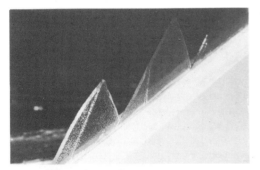

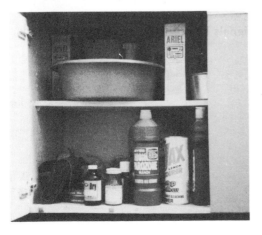

Falls account for about 40% of injuries at home to children aged under 5 years. Poisoning is the next most common cause, followed by cuts and bruises. Burns, scalds, choking, and suffocation are also important causes of injury or death. Some of these accidents can be prevented by better design or better components. The unsatisfactory design of windows above ground floor level shows the failure of designers to analyse safety requirements. They have not considered how to protect the youngest children, who are particularly likely to fall from windows. Windows should be inherently safe so that householders do not have to rely on safety devices which can (and often do) fail. Children climb on furniture and window ledges to see out, so the windowpane should be low enough for small children to see out of when they stand on the floor. The low-level window should be made of laminated safety glass so they cannot fall through it.

Unfortunately there is no requirement to use safety glass in windows or glass doors or partitions in the home. Children may easily run into glass doors, particularly if they are made of plain transparent glass with no markings; if the glass breaks the child may be severely injured by the razor-sharp edges.

The principle of prevention in other household accidents is to keep the child away from the hazard. Thus stairs should have gates to prevent toddlers falling down them and doors to balconies should be locked. Medicines, matches, and household chemicals such as bleach and white spirit should be locked away. Pills and other dangerous substances should be in childproof containers and never put in bottles or jars normally used for food or drink. Fires should be guarded, and parents need to be aware of how easily a child may be scalded by tipping over pans, kettles, and cups of hot liquid. Peanuts are a common cause of choking in young children, and children may suffocate themselves with plastic bags left lying around.

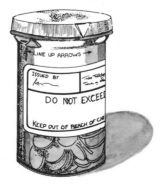

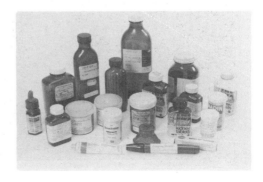

Accidents

Playground equipment injuries

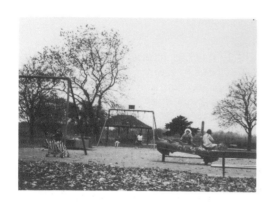

Injuries from playground equipment are often caused by the use of equipment in ways the designer did not envisage. It is dangerous for older children to use swings designed for younger ones or for several children to be on a swing at once. Children may fall or be pushed off a slide, especially when climbing up the slide while others are sliding down at the same time. Large rocking horses designed for several children to use at once may move too fast for the smaller ones, who may be thrown off. The long rocking horses are not suitable for the young children for whom they were not originally designed. It is difficult to design equipment which is completely safe without destroying the excitement which encourages children to use it. Children may get their arms or legs caught under playground roundabouts. Hazards of slides can be reduced by making the slide part of a grassy bank. Separation of age groups and more adult supervision would increase safety.

Environment

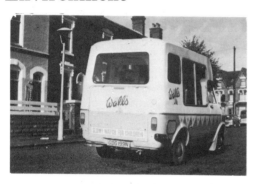

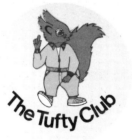

The Tufty Club

A kitchen window which looks into the garden improves safety. The lower branches of trees can be removed to prevent the tree being climbed. An ice cream van on the opposite side of a busy road can also be dangerous. Railways and canals are also hazards for children and it is difficult of make every stretch of water and rail childproof by walls and fences. These may be damaged by vandalism.

The Trident Trophy Scheme (open to secondary schools) encourages children to become proficient in survival, swimming, and lifesaving. The RoSPA has its own cycling proficiency scheme. Its safety education division has a Tufty Club, which caters primarily for children under 5 years. This is an association of some 14 000 local clubs, with perhaps 30–100 small children in each, and other children are enrolled as individuals. Most of these clubs are found in nursery schools, primary schools, and playgroups. They teach safety not only to young children but also to their parents. Other organisations helping in the promotion of safety education are the Health Education Council, the British Standards Institution, the Transport and Road Research Laboratory, the Medical Commission on Accident Prevention, the Fire Protection Association, and the Design Council.

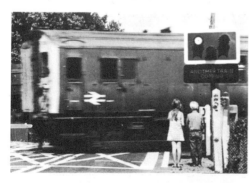

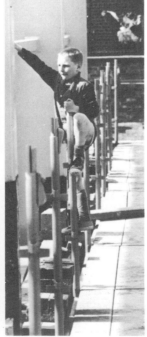

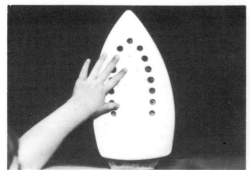

Doors to bathrooms and toilets should have handles that allow a bolted or locked door to be opened from the outside. Cooking stoves should be designed so that heated pots and pans as well as hot ovens are difficult for children to reach. Washing machines should stop automatically when the door is opened.

To be effective, protection must be provided for children of different ages and abilities. The toddler takes an overdose of medicine while exploring his environment, the 6 year old dashes into the road without realising the dangers, and the 12 year old falls while climbing a tree. The very young cannot be taught how to avoid these dangers and therefore must be protected from them. As children grow older their parents and teachers can teach them how to cope with dangerous situations such as roads, warn them of other dangers, and help them to assess what is a reasonable risk.

THE SEVERELY ILL CHILD

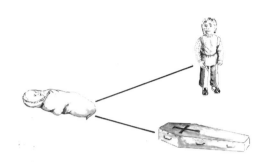

There is no precise definition of the severely ill child, but there are several conditions that need urgent treatment if he is to survive. In most cases the treatment will be started in the ambulance or the accident and emergency department. A glance at a child will show that he is desperately ill and that a rapid history and examination are needed. The time of onset and duration of the symptoms should be noted. Questions must include the presence of rash, occurrence of diarrhoea, vomiting, cough, or fast breathing. The child may be receiving drugs or have had access to tablets or household fluids. Recent loss of weight should be noted.

Examination

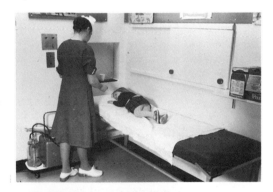

The first priority is to ensure a clear airway and adequate ventilation and circulation. The child needs to be nursed on his side as vomiting and aspiration are constant hazards. A suction pump with a catheter of adequate bore—for example, FG 14—should be kept next to the patient and turned on before examination begins. If the child is not breathing spontaneously 100% oxygen should be given with a closely fitting mask and Ambu, Penlon, or similar inflating bag. The child may usually be ventilated satisfactorily by this method and intubation can wait until an anaesthetist or member of the paediatric unit arrives. If he is breathing spontaneously 100% oxygen should be given by rubber funnel or a mask if the child can tolerate it.

Clinical signs of gross dehydration or a femoral pulse of poor volume indicates that the circulating blood volume is reduced and that intravenous fluids are required urgently. A low blood pressure indicates a severe reduction in plasma volume, but in children it is a late sign. Severe hypovolaemia may occur with no fall in the blood pressure. The child should be completely undressed and observed with good lighting.

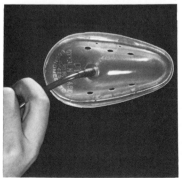
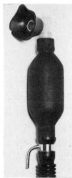

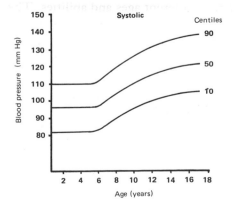

	Urgent investigations
Diabetes mellitus	BM stix, plasma glucose, urea, sodium, potassium, bicarbonate
Drowsiness after fit	
Head injury	
Poisons (including lead)	BM stix, analysis of vomitus, urine, blood
Septicaemia with meningitis or osteomyelitis	Blood culture, lumbar puncture
Gastroenteritis	BM stix, plasma sodium, potassium bicarbonate
Continuous convulsions	
Upper airway obstruction	
Bronchopneumonia	Chest x-ray
Bronchial asthma	
Bronchiolitis	Chest x-ray
Paroxysmal tachycardia	ECG
Peritonitis	Radiographs of abdomen

The severely ill child

Blood glucose test

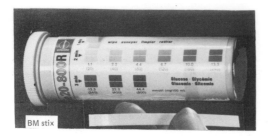

BM stix

A BM stix or similar strip test should be carried out before the physical examination. If the blood glucose concentration is more than 15 mmol/l (270 mg/100 ml) the child probably has diabetic ketoacidosis. If the blood glucose value is below 2·5 mmol/l (45 mg/100 ml) hypoglycaemia due to insulin overdose, salicylate poisoning, alcohol ingestion, or Reye's fatty liver syndrome should be considered.

Drowsiness and loss of consciousness

Fit

Head injury

Drugs

Septicaemia

±

Meningitis

If the child is drowsy or unconscious his parents should be questioned about the possibility of a recent fit, head injury, or drug ingestion. When urine from a child who has taken salicylates is tested with Phenistix the strip becomes brownish-red or purple. If the tablets were swallowed at least six hours earlier the absence of this colour change excludes salicylate poisoning. If there is any doubt plasma salicylate and barbiturate concentrations may need to be measured. Septicaemia does not produce specific signs, just a generally ill child, and there may be associated meningitis or osteomyelitis. Neck stiffness is often absent in infants with meningitis who are less than 2 years old. Urine should be kept for drug analysis.

The stomach contents should be aspirated to prevent accidental inhalation of gastric contents but an anaesthetist must be present during the procedure.

A severely dehydrated child has sunken eyes, a dry tongue, and inelastic skin and has usually not passed urine for several hours. The extent of recent weight loss may be known.

Acute gastroenteritis

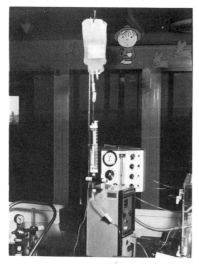

Acute gastroenteritis should be considered if there has been diarrhoea or vomiting. Infants may become severely ill before passing many loose stools, as there may be pooling of fluid in the gut. Rectal examination often produces a large amount of fluid stool. Intravenous fluids are needed urgently, preferably 0·45% sodium chloride with 2·5% glucose solution. The rate is 40 to 80 ml/kg body weight given over two to four hours. When urine has been passed the rate can be reduced and the solution changed to 0·18% sodium chloride with 4% glucose supplemented by potassium chloride 20 mmol/l. The aim is to complete rehydration 24 hours after admission, but if severe hypernatraemia is present rehydration is completed more slowly. The total volume required is the amount needed to make up the deficit added to the maintenance volumes. Severely dehydrated infants have a deficit of 10% of their body weight and moderately dehydrated infants 5% of the body weight.

In a severely shocked infant 10 ml of 0·9% sodium chloride solution or plasma for each kg of body weight should be given as quickly as possible by syringe intravenously using any large vein but preferably not the femoral vein.

Maintenance water requirements for 24 hours	
Age	Amount (ml/kg body weight)
1 week–6 months	150 ml
6 months–1 year	120 ml
1–3 years	100 ml
3–9 years	85 ml
9–12 years	70 ml
>12 years	60 ml

Diabetic ketoacidosis

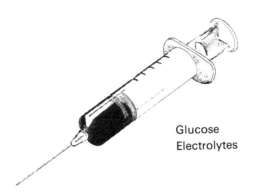

Glucose
Electrolytes

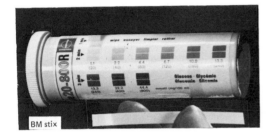

BM stix

If diabetic ketoacidosis is present (blood glucose concentration over 15 mmol/l (270 mg/100 ml)) intravenous 0·9% sodium chloride solution is needed urgently together with intravenous or intramuscular insulin. A senior member of the paediatric unit should be informed immediately but the intravenous fluid should be started in the accident and emergency department. There are often deep frequent respiratory movements due to metabolic acidosis. A 21-gauge butterfly needle can usually be inserted into a peripheral vein.

Plasma glucose, potassium, sodium, urea, and bicarbonate concentrations should be estimated on admission and at least at two and six hours after the beginning of treatment.

The initial intravenous fluid is 0·9% sodium chloride solution, which is given at a rate of 20 ml/kg body weight in the first 30 to 50 minutes. Many units no longer use sodium bicarbonate solution as the metabolic acidosis is corrected without it. Provided the plasma potassium concentration is not raised potassium chloride may be added to the bag of solution (20 mmol potassium chloride to every 500 ml of intravenous fluid) and the bag shaken thoroughly. The rate of infusing potassium chloride should be 0·1–0·2 mmol/kg/hour. Oral potassium supplements are given when the child can drink; a suitable dose is 0·5 g every eight hours. When the blood glucose concentration falls below 10 mmol/l (180 mg/100 ml) the fluid is changed to 0·18% sodium chloride with 4% glucose and supplementary potassium.

Insulin for initial treatment should always be the short-acting type, either soluble or neutral insulin. After a loading dose of 0·2 units/kg, 0·1 units/kg is given every hour until the blood glucose concentration, as shown by hourly BM stix tests, is less than 10 mmol/l (180 mg/100 ml). The dose of insulin is then reduced to 0·05 units/kg each hour. The same dose may be given as a continuous intravenous infusion using a syringe pump or by deep intramuscular injection. When the child is able to eat solid food (usually the next day) a subcutaneous injection of a short-acting insulin is given before each of the three main meals.

Acute gastric dilatation is common in severe ketosis and the stomach contents should be aspirated in a drowsy or unconscious patient to avoid aspiration pneumonia.

Convulsions

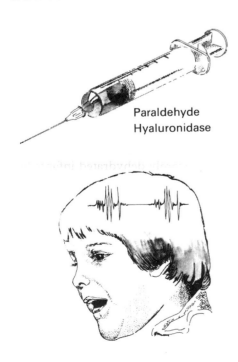

Paraldehyde
Hyaluronidase

Convulsions associated with fever occur in 3% of children aged 6 months to 5 years. Often there is no warning and the fever is not obvious to the mother. The child's clothes should be taken off and he should not be covered with a blanket. If the convulsions persist or start again, paraldehyde with hyaluronidase should be given intramuscularly. A glass syringe is ideal, but if only a plastic syringe is available the paraldehyde should be injected within two minutes of filling the syringe. If the convulsions do not stop within 10 minutes, the duty anaesthetist should be present while another drug is given intravenously. Diazepam must be given slowly over several minutes as there is a risk of respiratory arrest (see page 58 for further details).

Early transfer to the intensive care unit should be considered if a second dose of anticonvulsant is needed. Diazepam is extremely effective but it has been associated with respiratory arrest, especially when the patient has previously received barbiturate or the drug has been given too quickly. Standard solutions of diazepam cannot be diluted, which may lead to inaccuracy in measuring small doses. Inserting and holding the needle in the vein of a convulsing, fat toddler is often a difficult task. Diazepam is best used only by those experienced in intubating infants.

The severely ill child

Stridor

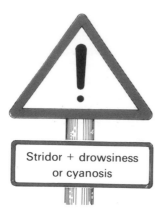

Stridor + drowsiness or cyanosis

Stridor with drowsiness is a dangerous combination of signs, and the duty anaesthetist should be called to the child immediately. Cyanosis is a terminal sign in these infants. The throat and mouth must not be examined nor a throat swab taken except by a skilled anaesthetist prepared to perform immediate intubation or tracheostomy if necessary. Although most patients with stridor have laryngitis, a few have epiglottitis or an inhaled foreign body, and an examination of the throat in these last two conditions may cause complete obstruction of the respiratory tract followed by cardiac arrest. The child should be admitted to the intensive care unit or taken directly to the operating theatre as urgent intubation by a skilled anaesthetist may be required.

Raised respiratory rate

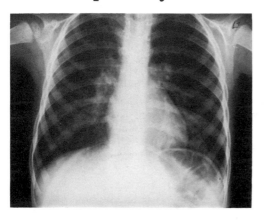

A raised respiratory rate at rest suggests pneumonia or peritonitis. Staphylococcal pneumonia may make the child extremely ill because of the associated septicaemia. Pneumonia causes the alae nasi to move actively and there may be a cough, fever, and adventitious sounds in the chest.

Infants with bronchiolitis may deteriorate suddenly and a rasping cough and recession of the chest wall may be the main features.

If there was choking just before the dyspnoea began the possibility of an inhaled foreign body must be considered.

When an enlarged liver accompanies a raised respiratory rate congestive cardiac failure is present. If there is no cardiac murmur, paroxysmal supraventricular tachycardia should be considered.

Abdominal tenderness

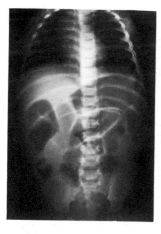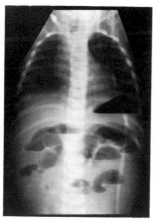

Generalised abdominal tenderness suggests peritonitis, which may be due to perforation of the appendix or of the small gut after intestinal obstruction. An obstructed inguinal hernia is a form of intestinal obstruction which is easily missed. In suspected intestinal obstruction urgent radiographs should be taken in the supine and erect positions to show fluid levels in distended loops of small gut. Fluid levels are also found in children with gastroenteritis but are present in the large gut as well as the small intestine. If the patient cannot stand erect similar information can be obtained from radiographs taken using a horizontal beam with the patient lying on his side.

Rash

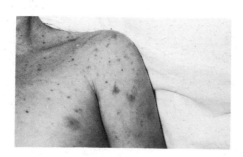

If there is a generalised purpuric rash—on the trunk as well as the neck (which does not disappear when pressure is applied)—a presumptive diagnosis of meningococcal septicaemia should be made.

Blood should be taken for culture, and, using the same needle in the vein, 0·5 megaunit (300 mg) of benzylpenicillin is given slowly intravenously. The same dose is given irrespective of age. Children may die within a few hours of the onset of this disease and urgent treatment is necessary.

DEVELOPMENT AT 18 MONTHS

18 months	Normal	Doubtful	Abnormal
Alertness			
Pincer grip			
Right			
Left			
Simple commands			
Standing			
Walking			
2-cube tower			

During the second year infants begin to walk and talk. Mobility enables them to explore the shapes and textures of objects in their environment but brings with it the dangers of swallowing or aspirating objects they find. These activities enable them to wean themselves from close maternal attachment, and this process is sometimes accompanied by rebellion against the mother.

History

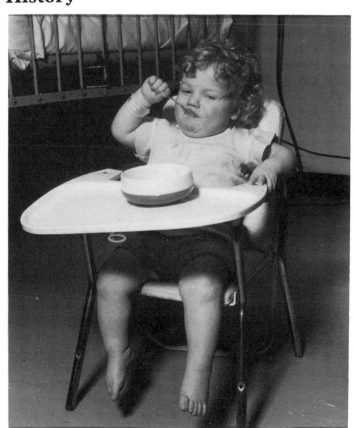

The mother should be asked whether she has any problems and whether the child has had any illnesses since the previous visit. She should be asked when he started to stand, walk, and feed himself with a spoon and drink from a cup. The number of words he says with meaning is noted.

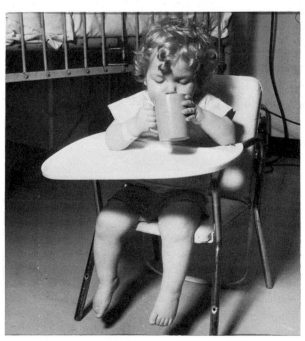

Development at 18 months

Walking

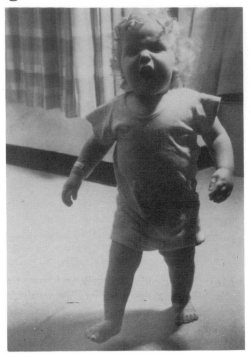

Nearly all infants will be walking by the age of 18 months. An exception are those who were "bottom-shufflers"; since they already move around fast on their bottoms they tend to learn to walk later than average. Other infants who are not walking by this age should be seen every two months and if they are not walking by the age of 2 years they should be seen by a developmental specialist.

When walking begins there is a wide gait and the toes often point outwards or inwards. Occasionally infants start walking on their toes, but within a month the whole sole should be on the ground. Some infants fear letting go of a hand but may become independent by being allowed to push a toy pram or a wheeled toy. The infant will enjoy taking the pots and pans out of the cupboard, and the provision of a special cupboard to do this will encourage him.

Language

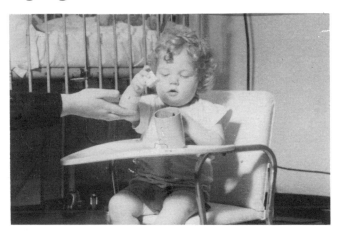

Words are only the final stage in the development of language, and the ability to communicate is more important than the number of words a child can say distinctly. He should be able to obey simple commands—to take an object out of a cup and give it to his mother or to put it into the cup—and failure to communicate in this or in similar ways is abnormal. Long babbled conversations which are unintelligible are normal and are called jargon.

He enjoys looking at simple picture books and points at objects in them with his finger. He starts showing his independence, albeit capriciously, by refusing certain foods or refusing to conform to his mother's wishes.

Manipulation

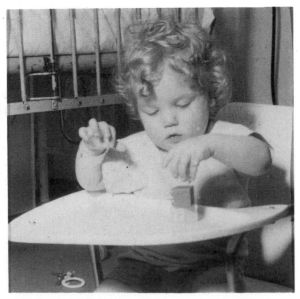

About this time the child will start to help to take off his shoes and socks and become aware of the different parts of his body. He can feed himself with a spoon without tipping the food all over the table. He sees and picks up small objects with his thumb and index finger (pincer grip). He is able to build one-inch cubes into a tower of two or three provided he has had previous experience of trying to do it.

Inability to stand by himself or lack of a pincer grip in each hand are indications for referral to a developmental specialist. Failure to make spontaneous sounds or to obey simple commands is another indication that further advice is needed.

DEVELOPMENT AT 2 YEARS

2 years	Normal	Doubtful	Abnormal
Alertness or interest			
Number of words			
2-word phrases			
Walking			
Miniatures			
6-cube tower			

Most 2 year olds can walk and run as well as climb up and down stairs. They mimic activities, understand symbols, and have an independent spirit.

History

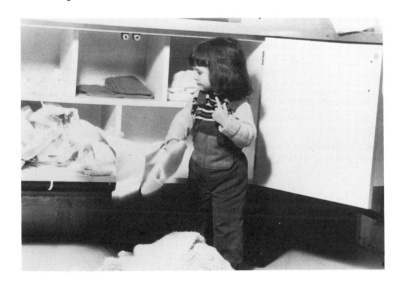

The mother should be asked whether the child has had any illnesses since the previous visit and whether she has any problems. The date he began to walk without help is noted and whether he says two-word phrases. If he does not speak more than a few words she should be asked whether he obeys simple commands. She is also asked whether he feeds himself with a spoon or a cup without spilling and how much he helps with dressing.

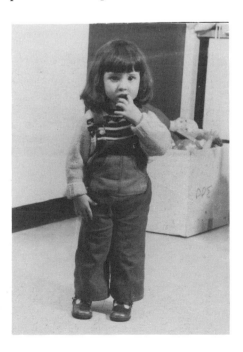

Examination

His steadiness in walking, symmetry of gait, and distance between his feet during walking are noted.

If the child makes short, clear two-word phrases this suggests that his speech and hearing are normal. He should be able to identify four parts of his body when asked in a soft voice.

Development at 2 years

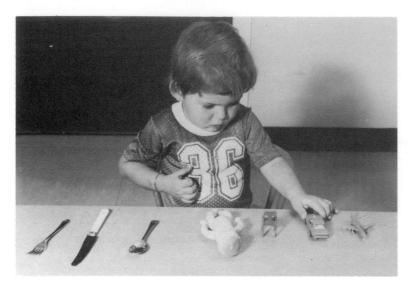

He can usually build a tower of six cubes, and ataxia, tremor, or clumsiness could be noted during this attempt. He turns the pages of a book singly and will name some of the objects in a simple book. He can be given miniatures and will show that he understands their function. A girl will play at making tea and a boy needs no encouragement to push a small car across the table. A miniature chair is placed on the table by the child in a position which shows that he understands its function.

Vision can be tested by showing him miniature toys, held 10 feet away from him, and asking him to match them with corresponding toys of normal size on the table in front of him or to name them. The test should be given to each eye separately using a plastic eye shield or bandage.

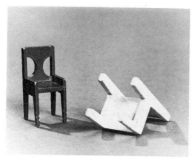
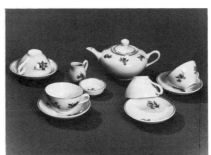
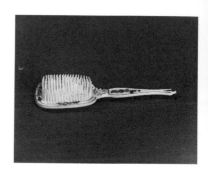

Indications for referral

Failure to walk

Lack of interest

< 5 words

Each of the following is an indication for referral to a developmental specialist: failure to walk independently, complete lack of interest in the test objects, lack of two-word phrases, and inability to say more than five words. Strabismus or absence of pincer grip should have been detected at earlier examinations.

THE HANDICAPPED CHILD

	Rate per 1000 children
Mental handicap	30
Cerebral palsy	3
Epilepsy	6
Asthma	100
Blindness	0·25
Squint	30
Refractive error	50
Hearing defects	
Mild, usually due to glue ear	50
Moderate (need hearing aid)	2
Severely deaf	1

The parents of a child who may be abnormal will want to know what is wrong, the treatment required, the prognosis, and the chances that a future child will have a similar problem. The experience of managing handicap or chronic disability will vary from doctor to doctor. Although about 10% of preschool children in a general practice have a chronic disability most have asthma or behaviour disorders. Nevertheless, there are many more children who may be brought by parents worried about developmental variations and learning difficulties, and a general practitioner can help parents considerably if he has an interest in and experience of the normal range of abilities.

A general practitioner is likely to see one new case of Down syndrome every 10 years. A district unit for the assessment and care of handicapped children may have about 60 with cerebral palsy and 80 with mental retardation without cerebral palsy attending the centre.

About one in 1000 children have severe hearing loss and are managed mainly at special centres, but many children in every general practice have fluctuating or persistent hearing loss due to secretory otitis media. Severe visual defects are often associated with other abnormalities, but defects in visual acuity which could be corrected by spectacles often pass undetected for long periods. Although a family doctor may have only two children with epilepsy in his practice a consultant paediatrician may be following up about 50 in the general outpatient clinics.

Chronic handicaps affecting the central nervous system or special senses are rare in general practice; they are not simply medical problems and for adequate assessment need the help of workers from several disciplines, including social and educational. Most of these children are now referred to their local district paediatrician. This group will be discussed in detail because management illustrates important aspects of child care.

Discovery

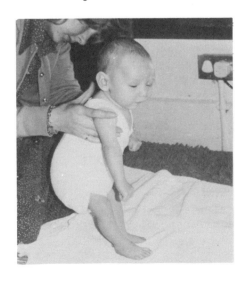

Abnormalities may be noted at birth—for example, Down syndrome or myelomeningocele. A neighbour, relative, or friend may notice that an infant is not performing like her own child of that age and may point it out to the mother. A doctor may discover that the child has developmental delay at a routine assessment clinic, during a consultation for an acute illness, or while following up children of low birth weight. The mother may have read books on child development and realise that her child is not behaving normally. Unless a doctor discovers the disability there may be a considerable delay before the mother summons up the courage to seek appropriate advice. Mothers may raise questions with their health visitor when she visits the home or at the clinic, and health visitors play an important part in encouraging mothers to report their fears and in arranging referrals. If the mother suspects that her child is abnormal she should be referred to a consultant paediatrician or a senior clinical medical officer with special experience in assessing handicap. Mothers are usually correct in their assessment. Once a mother has shown this initiative any delay may make her distrust later medical advice.

The handicapped child

First consultation

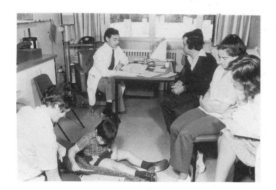

Patients are referred to consultant paediatricians by family doctors, but the new consultant paediatrician with a special interest in the community (community paediatrician) or senior clinical medical officer receives some referrals from health visitors or community clinics by agreement with family doctors. The family is seen by the consultant alone at the first visit, or at most by three members of the staff (consultant, psychologist, and physiotherapist), as the presence of a large team may prevent the mother from expressing her worries. After taking the history and examining the child the doctor should tell the parents the possible diagnosis. He should explain that this is a provisional diagnosis and that relevant blood, urine, or radiographic tests will be carried out and assessments performed by various members of the staff in the day care unit. These results will be discussed with the parents in the presence of all the therapists at the second visit, so that a programme of management can be agreed.

Assessment and treatment

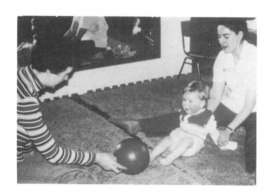

The appropriate members of the team can then be selected and asked to see the child before the second visit. Most of the children will need to be seen by an ophthalmologist and also need a hearing test. Only a minority need the opinion of a neurologist. As the physiotherapist, occupational therapist, and speech therapist often assess a child together they learn part of each other's jobs and can advise whether help from another discipline is indicated. Therapists often take two to three hours to assess a child, taking the opportunity to assess him during a meal and at play as well as by formal tests. Assessing patients without having a part in their further management can be frustrating for therapists, but they are seeing more patients in their own homes, nurseries, and schools to advise on practical management. Formal exercises in hospital are avoided and an attempt is made to teach mothers, nursery supervisors, and teachers how to help the child. A community occupational therapist who also has a session in hospital may help considerably. Taking children out of school for treatment in hospital has the disadvantage of accentuating the stigma of being different.

Second consultation

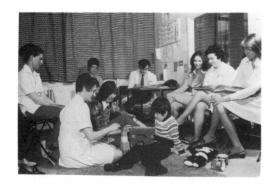

Just before the family is seen on the second visit the therapists and consultant meet to plan the child's management. A "key worker" should be selected to avoid duplicating treatment and give the parents a person to latch on to and telephone in a crisis. The whole team then sits down with the parents and the consultant discusses the diagnosis, management, and prognosis. If the family's health visitor also attends with the parents she can reinforce and explain at subsequent home visits what the hospital team discussed. She can also provide the hospital workers with an insight into family dynamics. The parents should be given an ample opportunity to discuss their worries and they often bring a list, which saves forgetting important points. Some parents may wish to discuss these points with the consultant alone as they may be intimidated by the large team.

In some units the medical social worker sees the parents between the two visits but in others she sees them at the second visit or afterwards. Most families with handicapped children need social work support at some stage. All parents should be offered a consultation with a geneticist even if they are not contemplating a new pregnancy in the near future.

Parental reactions

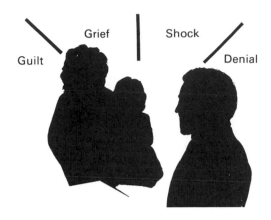

Guilt Grief Shock Denial

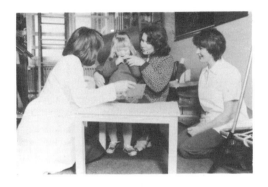

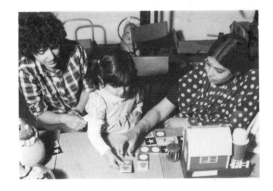

Initially young parents or parents of first-born children may have difficulty in persuading a doctor that the child is abnormal. This may delay the diagnosis or cause frustration and considerable subsequent hostility to all medical advisers. Parents deserve to know the truth about their child and all aspects of the prognosis should be discussed honestly. Most parents are shocked when the diagnosis is discussed and feel detached. The reality of the symptoms may be denied, the doctor's competence questioned, and the parents may search for an alternative opinion. Both parents should be present when the diagnosis is explained so that they can support each other. They usually need to be seen again shortly afterwards because they may be too stunned at the initial interview to understand what is being discussed and may later deny that important aspects were mentioned at all. Many units give the parents a written summary of the findings and programme of management, which may be the same or a simplified version of the summary provided for the family doctor. Details of the 1981 Education Act are given on page 102.

The parents become increasingly dispirited and lacking in self-confidence and mourn for the normal child they have lost. They may blame themselves for the child's problems and feel guilty about their inability to protect him from the event or come to terms with reality. Some parents deny the diagnosis for some time but others continue to do so for several years. Some become unable to understand anything but the simplest information.

Both parents may develop symptoms of grief: depression, sighing, crying, preoccupation with the child, loss of appetite, and sleep problems. Often these symptoms lead to irritablity and the parents may be hostile towards the child, the medical staff caring for him, and even their other children. The other children may develop behaviour problems because their parents appear remote and uncaring. The health visitor may be able to help the parents come to terms with their anger and denial because she is already familiar to the parents and so may avoid the hostility which the parents may feel towards the hospital staff who have diagnosed the handicap.

Training junior staff in the management of handicapped children is difficult. Most registrars can see a child only over a year, and families usually need support for much longer. Confidence in the doctor and ability to discuss problems with him is attained only after a long period and is not easily transferred.

Early and appropriate treatment helps to support the parents and is therefore indirectly beneficial to the child. More research is needed to determine the effects of various treatments on the long-term prognosis. Research is also needed into the effects of the treatments provided by physiotherapists, occupational therapists, speech therapists, social workers, and child psychiatrists, so that they may use their resources rationally. At present some of their work is interchangeable.

Parents' groups

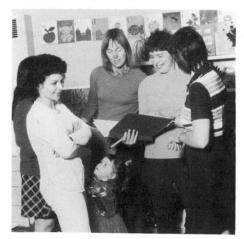

There are several associations of parents of children with various handicapping diseases and many have local branches. Most associations raise money for research and enable parents with children with similar problems to make best use of local resources and discuss mutual problems. Social workers usually have a list of the addresses of local groups. Some groups are arranged by the social services department in each district and may be organised by a social worker with the help of an occupational therapist or physiotherapist.

The handicapped child

Education

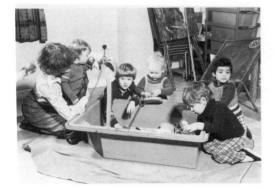

For preschool children with handicaps the opportunity playgroup has great advantages. Up to a third of the children are handicapped and the rest normal. Children with and without handicaps can mix, and the parents of handicapped children are brought together for mutual support. These groups have a high staff to child ratio, and an occupational therapist or physiotherapist should have a regular commitment to advise on the management of handicapped children. The object is to enable the child to reach his maximum potential and to enable him to attend the most suitable local school. Close observation in this setting, a knowledge of local facilities, formal testing by an educational psychologist, and discussion with the parents will help to make the transition to a school. Local education authorities have to provide some form of education for handicapped children from the age of 2 years and to provide the necessary transport.

Most children with handicaps will go to normal primary schools and an increasing number with learning problems will also go there. For example, children with Down syndrome always used to go to special schools, but a few are being admitted to normal primary schools. This requires more staff with special training and abilities together with extra facilities for small classes. Some education authorities find it difficult to find the extra resources or change staff attitudes.

Regional centres

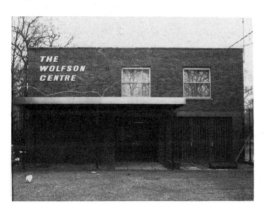

Regional centres for the assessment and care of the handicapped have many advantages, including the ready availability of paediatric ophthalmologists, neurologists, and ENT and orthopaedic surgeons. But parents may find it difficult to travel to a regional centre often. The strengths and weaknesses of local facilities for treating and educating handicapped children are usually known best by the paediatricians and senior clinical medical officers working locally. If they are in clinical charge of the patient they are likely to press for the provision of local services. Assessment without appropriate care increases the frustration of parents with a handicapped child.

SCHOOL FAILURE

Children have to go to school whether they like it or not. Parents must by law ensure that their children are educated between the ages of 5 and 16, and local education authorities have a duty to provide appropriate schools and teachers. The Education Act 1981 laid down the duty of local education authorities to discover children with special educational needs by reason of learning difficulties and to provide appropriate help. School governors and head teachers also have duties to ensure that children's special educational needs are known to staff. Many children do not find school unpleasant, but for some it is a miserable experience. A few cannot bear to leave home while others just dislike school or are unhappy there. Although teachers try to treat children as individuals and provide appropriate learning experiences at a pace suited to their needs, the sheer size of the task means that much teaching is carried out in groups and individual help is limited. The child who fails to learn with his group may get extra help but unless he can make up ground he may find himself habitually failing. Few people enjoy failing all the time and a child who has no option but to attend school may react to failure in several ways. He may remove himself from the situation by playing truant or becoming withdrawn and "switching off"; conversely, he may protest by drawing attention to himself through aggressive or destructive behaviour or by clowning.

There are many reasons why children fail at school, including poor teaching, but some of the commonest may be explored by the family doctor who is approached by anxious parents.

Truanting

Switching off

Aggression

Destructiveness

Clowning

Absence from school

Teachers try to help children to acquire the basic skills in a logical, progressive sequence. A child who is often absent from school may have great difficulty in filling in the gaps. Continual short absences may prove more damaging educationally than a few prolonged absences because teachers may not realise that the child is missing a lot of schooling. If they do recognise the loss they can try to cover lost ground. It is important to try to discover how much school a child is missing and why. The child may genuinely be often unwell but he may also complain of feeling unwell because of anxiety.

	28 Sept 81						6 Oct 81				
	M	T	W	T	F		M	T	W	T	F
Amis D	✓	✓	✓	✓	✓		✓	✓	✓	✓	✓
Appleby C	✓	✓	✓	✓	✓		✓	✓	✓	✓	✓
Brown J	✓	✓	✓	✓	✓		✓	✓	✓	✓	✓
Brown S		O	O	O	O	✓		O	O	O	O	✓
Burridge H	✓	✓	✓		O	✓		✓	✓	✓	✓	✓
Collins A	✓	✓	✓	✓	✓		✓	✓	✓	✓	✓
Clipper C	✓	✓	✓	✓	✓		✓	✓	✓	✓	✓
Chatham B	✓	✓	✓	✓	✓		✓	✓	✓	✓	✓
Davidson W	✓	✓	✓				✓	✓	✓	✓	✓
David W	✓	✓	✓				✓	✓	✓	✓	✓
Dee L	✓			O	✓		O	✓			✓
Dunster W		O	O	O	O	O	✱	O	O	O	O	✓
Dwight J	✓		✓	✓	✓	✓		✓	✓	✓	✓	✓
Exbridge L		O	O	O	O	O	✱	O	O	✓		O	O
Frothingham P	✓	✓	✓	✓	✓		✓	✓	✓	✓	✓
Harcourt J	✓	✓	✓	✓	✓		✓	✓	✓	✓	✓
Johns W	✓	✓	✓	✓	✓		✓	✓	✓	✓	✓
Jones P	✓	✓	✓		✓		✓	✓	✓	✓	✓
Jones A	✓	✓	✓	✓	✓		✓	✓	✓	✓	✓
Lappet B		O	O	O	O	O	✱	O	✓		O	O	✓
Lumps C	✓	✓	✓	✓	✓		✓	✓	✓	✓	✓

School failure

Physical and sensory difficulties

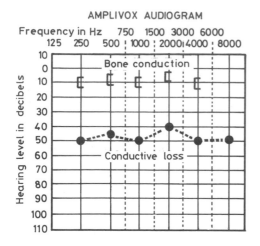

AMPLIVOX AUDIOGRAM

Frequency in Hz
125 250 500 750 1000 1500 2000 3000 4000 6000 8000

Hearing level in decibels
10
0
10
20
30
40
50
60
70
80
90
100
110

Bone conduction

Conductive loss

Although each child is given a medical examination before or on school entry and has his vision and hearing checked, it is still possible to miss, for example, a fluctuating conductive hearing loss. Concerned parents are good observers of their children and it is worth questioning them about any difficulties they have noticed at particular times or in particular circumstances. Some children who attend school regularly may be unwell while they are there and therefore unable to concentrate on what is happening.

Intellectual difficulties

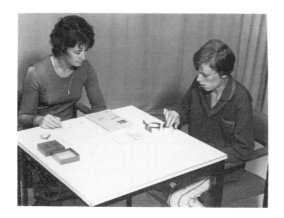

Teachers do not expect all children to learn at the same pace but some children are much slower than those at the slow end of a fairly wide normal range. Not all schools make special provision for slow learners, but without some extra or separate teaching they may be unable to cope. The school itself may have recognised the problem and asked the parents' consent to refer the child to the school psychological service for advice. The service, run by the local education authority, usually accepts referrals from any source, so general practitioners and parents may make a direct approach if they wish.

Developmental delay and specific learning difficulties

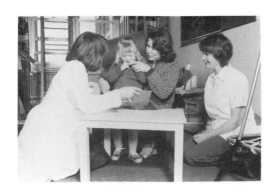

It is not easy to decide whether a child's development is at the slower end of normal limits or whether there is a more serious problem. Parents are particularly concerned about slow language development. A referral to a speech therapist should help in making a differential diagnosis between delay and specific problems in language development.

While not unintelligent, some children have great difficulty in mastering the basic skills of literacy and numeracy, despite regular teaching. There is disagreement over the use of the term "dyslexia" to describe a specific reading disability, because of the problems of both definition and causation. Some severely handicapped readers have spatial and sequencing difficulties while others find it hard to perceive and analyse sounds in words. The diagnosis of specific learning difficulties in basic skills is a complex process and help should be sought from an educational psychologist and a skilled remedial teacher.

Emotional difficulties

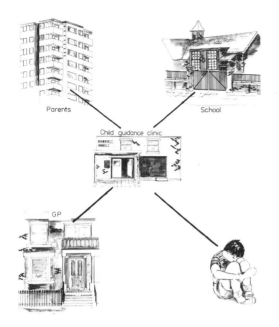

A child who is failing in circumstances from which there is no legal escape will usually react in some way, so most children who do badly at school will have accompanying emotional stress. For some children, however, school failure may be the outcome of personal emotional difficulties with family relationships and the child's social environment. The child who is overprotected and the child who is rejected may each fail in school and may produce physical as well as emotional symptoms of stress.

Where severe emotional difficulties are suspected referral to the local child guidance clinic is appropriate. The team, which usually includes a child psychiatrist and an educational psychologist, is well placed to liaise between general practitioners, the parents, the child, and the school and can organise help for the child.

MINOR ORTHOPAEDIC PROBLEMS

In-toeing

Bow legs

Knock knees

Flat feet

Minor orthopaedic problems such as in-toeing, bow legs, knock knees, and flat feet cause anxiety to both parents and doctors.

In-toeing is nearly always due to one of three conditions: metatarsus varus, which affects the foot; medial tibial torsion, which affects the lower leg; and persistent femoral anteversion, which affects the whole leg. In managing all these minor orthopaedic anomalies the whole child must be examined to ensure that the orthopaedic problem is not part of a more serious generalised disorder.

Metatarsus varus or adductus

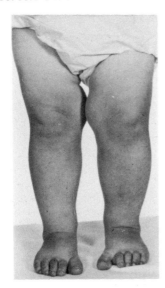 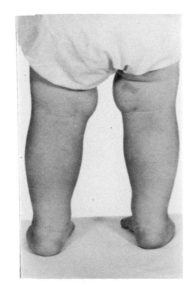

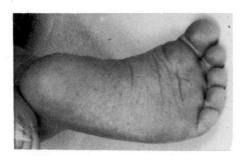

Metatarsus varus or adductus, hookfoot or skewfoot, is very common. It may be noticed at or soon after birth but is most obvious and causes most anxiety when the child starts to walk. At this stage the child falls frequently. Parents often ascribe the falls to the pronounced in-toeing rather than to the complex problem of learning bipedal gait. Metatarsus varus can be distinguished from talipes equino varus as only the forefoot is abnormal. The heel is in line with the leg and the foot can be flexed to 90° or more.

Ninety per cent of all cases of metatarsus varus correct spontaneously without treatment by the age of 3 to 4 years. Most of the remaining children will have no complaints about their feet; a few will show persistent deformity, which will require treatment by plasters and occasionally surgery. When advising parents to wait for natural resolution in the face of obvious deformity it is important to explain three things: firstly, the natural history and high spontaneous recovery rate; secondly, the time recovery is likely to take; and thirdly, that if their child is the "odd man out" who does not correct then adequate and full correction is possible and has not been jeopardised by waiting.

Medial tibial torsion

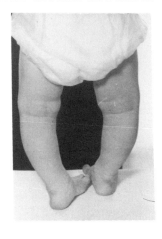
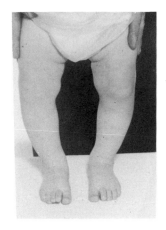

Medial tibial torsion is nearly always associated with outward curving of the tibia, which is an exaggeration of the normal or physiological bowing of the tibia. In medial tibial torsion when the knee is pointing forwards the foot is medially rotated 20°–30° whereas in the adult the foot is normally rotated outwards 0°–25°. Both the medial torsion and the bowing should correct spontaneously by the age of 3 to 4 years provided they are not associated with any other abnormality. No special shoes or splints are necessary. Beware of marked unilateral bowing, which suggests an epiphyseal abnormality.

Tibia vara and rickets

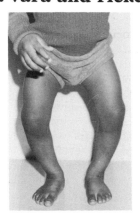
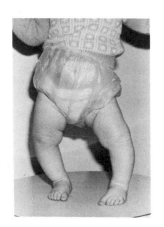

Tibia vara, due to epiphyseal growth abnormality, should be considered, particularly in West Indian and West African children, if the bowing is very pronounced and the angulation immediately below the knee.

Dietary rickets should also be considered, particularly among immigrant children with pronounced bowing of the tibiae. Swelling round the knees, wrists, and ankles, craniotabes, Harrison's sulcus, and a "rachitic rosary" should also be looked for.

Persistent femoral anteversion and retroversion

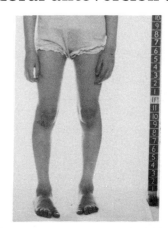

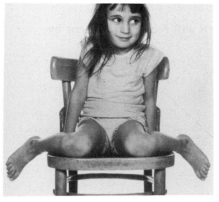
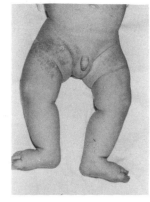

In persistent femoral anteversion the whole leg turns in from the hip. The patellae look towards each other—so-called squinting patellae. The child characteristically sits between the legs. To demonstrate the femoral neck anteversion the child should be examined with the hips extended and the knees flexed. Internal rotation of the hip is greater than external rotation and can easily be seen and measured. In 80% of these children the anteversion will correct by the age of 8 years. It is doubtful whether any form of special shoe or splint can influence the condition. If there is severe persistent functional and cosmetic deformity after the age of 8 femoral osteotomy is occasionally indicated.

Femoral retroversion (out-toeing) is the opposite condition. The child lies or stands with the legs externally rotated 90°. There is often no internal rotation in extension at the hip. This condition corrects within a year of the child starting to walk. It is important to check the extent of abduction in flexion of the hips carefully as congenital dislocation of the hip can also cause external rotation.

Minor orthopaedic problems

Knock knees

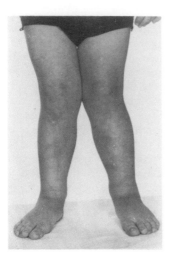

Seventy-five per cent of children aged 2 to $4\frac{1}{2}$ years have some degree of intermalleolar separation. Up to $3\frac{1}{2}$ inches (9 cm) measured with the child lying down is acceptable. There is no evidence that shoe modification, splints, or exercises affect this condition. It is important to look for pronounced asymmetry, short stature, and other skeletal abnormalities which may indicate a more serious problem. If the intermalleolar is more than $3\frac{1}{2}$ inches an AP radiograph of both legs on the same film is probably the most useful radiological investigation as it will not only show the knee deformity but also the hip and ankle joints and the whole of the long bones of the lower limbs on one film. If the condition does not correct spontaneously medial epiphyseal stapling at 10 to 11 years or corrective osteotomy at maturity is the treatment of choice.

Flat feet

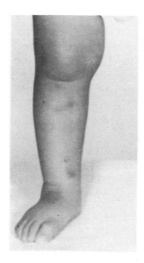

There are two forms of flat feet: the first group are pain free and have normal mobility and normal muscle power, and the second are painful, stiff, or hypermobile and show abnormal muscle power—that is, are weak or spastic. The simplest method of testing is to ask the patient to stand on tiptoe. If the arches are restored by this simple test then the feet are almost certainly normal.

It is important to remember that the normal foot is flat when the child starts to stand. The medial arch does not develop until the second or third year of life. Most children with flat feet will fall into the first group. These characteristics are commonly familial or racial. Treatment with insoles, shoe modification, or exercises is unlikely to make any difference to the shape of the feet. Shoe wear can be a problem and insoles or medial stiffening may help. Surgery is rarely indicated. The second group is important as there is either a local bony or inflammatory problem in the foot that needs diagnosis and treatment or the flat foot is part of a more generalised condition such as severe generalised joint laxity, cerebral palsy, peroneal spastic flat foot, or Down syndrome.

Joint laxity

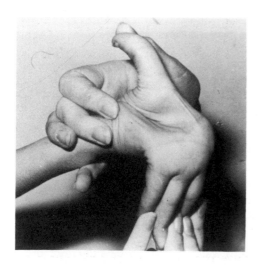

Joint laxity should always be considered in children with a clumsy or awkward gait. The presence of three or more of the following are evidence of definite joint laxity: in the arm, hyperextension of the wrist and metacarpophalangeal joints, the thumb, or the elbow; in the leg, hyperextension of the knee or ankle. Laxity is frequently familial or it may be part of a generalised disorder such as osteogenesis imperfecta, Ehlers–Danlos syndrome, or Marfan's syndrome.

When counselling parents about minor orthopaedic problems it is important to examine the patient fully, to explain the natural history of the condition, and to check carefully for more serious disorders.

LIMP

The child with a limp may have a minor injury which will recover spontaneously in a few hours or a condition which may affect him for life if treatment is delayed. A diagnosis must be made, or if this is not possible the child should be observed in hospital until he has fully recovered. A full history and careful examination of the whole child is essential. A radiograph of the affected area is taken, but pain in the thigh referred from the hip can lead to the wrong area being examined. Parents' observations may sometimes sound odd but should not be dismissed. Abnormal physical signs are usually present in any child with a limp which has a serious cause. Limp may be due to pain, leg inequality, neuromuscular dysfunction, or rarely, psychological disturbance. These groups often overlap.

Pain

Leg inequality

Neuromuscular dysfunction

Psychological disturbance

Pain

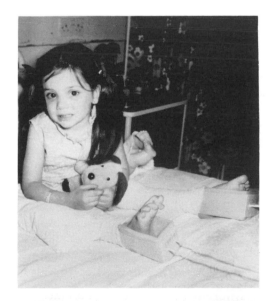

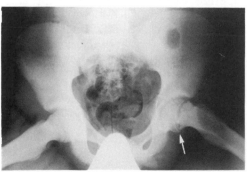

The commonest cause of limp is pain. Injury may produce muscle strain or fractures but non-accidental injury or foreign body should always be considered. Any pain which does not settle within a few days or recurs should be investigated. Perthes's disease, slipped upper femoral epiphysis, and benign tumours such as osteoid osteoma often produce intermittent pain, which can easily be dismissed as a recurrent muscle strain.

Transient synovitis (observation hip, coxalgia fugax) is a common condition of unknown cause. The child suddenly starts limping and there is spasm of the hip muscles but no other abnormal signs. He may have a mild fever and raised erythrocyte sedimentation rate. Transient synovitis usually settles with a short period of bed rest. Traction is helpful to relieve muscle spasm and pain. Most children have no further problems, but a few may have recurrent attacks and subsequently develop changes of Perthes's disease or juvenile arthritis. It is important to eliminate more serious conditions such as septic arthritis or osteomyelitis, Perthes's disease, juvenile chronic arthritis, slipped upper femoral epiphysis (which is outside the age group of this book), and tuberculosis.

Septic arthritis—The child with septic arthritis is usually seriously ill but beware of the child suffering from immune deficiency, immune suppression, or who has been given a short course of antibiotics which mask the signs and symptoms. Perthes's disease and slipped upper femoral epiphysis should be seen on a radiograph. It is important to take a frog lateral view as well as an anteroposterior view of the hips to diagnose and evaluate these two conditions. Juvenile chronic arthritis and tuberculosis are likely to have a longer time course and also show radiographic changes.

Limp

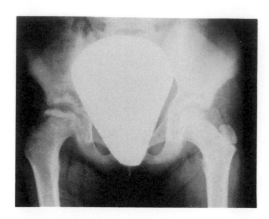

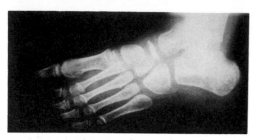

Perthes's disease—Treatment for Perthes's disease is confusing both to the general practitioner and the orthopaedic surgeon. There is evidence which suggests that Perthes's disease is due to temporary ischaemia of the femoral head. Treatment cannot prevent the disease but is aimed at improving the outcome. Many patients need no treatment after the acute episode of pain and spasm. Regular radiographic monitoring of the hip is necessary to ensure that the femoral head remains within the acetabulum. If the femoral head begins to move out of the acetabulum abduction splints, plasters, or surgery may be needed to achieve containment of the head.

Osteochondroses—Osteochondritis of the tarsal navicular may cause pain over the medial arch of the foot. A radiograph will confirm the diagnosis. Most cases settle with reduction of activity. Sometimes a short period in a below-knee plaster is necessary. Osteochondritis affecting the heel or the tibial tubercle and osteochondritis dissecans of the knee rarely occur in this age group.

Verrucas, foreign bodies, and minor fractures may also cause pain in the foot. Persistent swelling, particularly around the ankle, suggests juvenile chronic arthritis, which commonly presents in the foot in children.

In this age group pain around the knee is uncommon although it becomes increasingly common in early adolescence. Causes of pain in the knee include bone and joint sepsis, chronic inflammatory conditions, and mechanical derangement such as a discoid meniscus.

Leg inequality

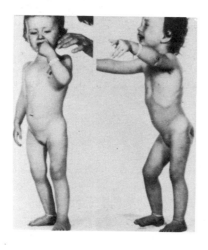

A short leg must be distinguished from apparent shortening due to pelvic obliquity, scoliosis, or joint deformity. Congenital defects such as short femur or tibia are usually obvious. Despite early screening programmes congenital dislocation of the hip must always be considered. Typically the leg is short and externally rotated, and abduction in flexion is limited. The child usually walks with the leg straight on the dislocated side and the knee flexed on the normal side. The doctor may consider that the flexed knee is abnormal and fail to recognise that the opposite hip is abnormal. Hemiplegic cerebral palsy, spinal dysraphism, and poliomyelitis cause poor growth of the affected leg and can be detected by a neurological examination. The whole spine should be examined for the warning signs of dysraphism: a naevus, hairy patch, pit, or lipoma. Epiphyseal injury from trauma or sepsis can cause shortening deformity.

Neuromuscular and hysterical disorders

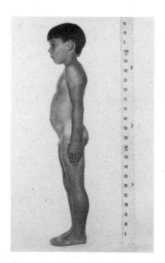

Complex disturbances of gait, such as incoordination or weakness due to cerebral palsy, muscular dystrophy, or spinal or cerebral tumour, may be described by the parents as a limp. A careful history and examination will usually suggest the diagnosis.

If a limp has an emotional origin diagnosis may be difficult. Usually the pattern of gait is bizarre and the physical signs inconsistent. It is essential to eliminate any possible organic cause. Often it is necessary to admit the patient to hospital for a few days' observation. A bone scan is a most useful investigation both to eliminate the possibility of abnormality in the bone which has not been detected by radiographs and to show up hot or cold areas before radiographic changes are present.

SERVICES FOR CHILDREN: PRIMARY CARE

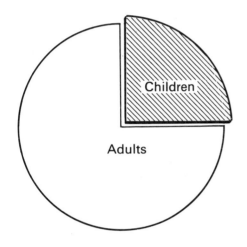

The general practitioner provides continuous care for the whole family, and his intimate knowledge of the fears and aspirations of each individual enables him to act as a trusted counsellor in both preventive and curative medicine. Specialists in the community or hospital provide the support he requests. About 25% of the work of the general practitioner concerns children, and he recognises that their needs are different from those of patients in other age groups because they are both dependent and developing.

Unfortunately, the primary care of children is still divided: general practitioners provide a mainly treatment service (for those who seek it) while the clinical medical officers of the child health and school health services provide a surveillance, prevention, and health education service. General practitioners are performing an increasing amount of preventive work stimulated by the report *Healthier Children—Thinking Prevention* from the Royal College of General Practitioners in 1982.

Practice organisation

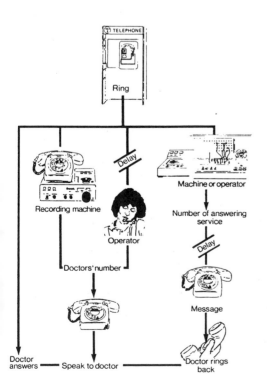

Illness in children often starts suddenly and arouses acute anxiety in parents. Practice receptionists need to appreciate this natural protective response and allow children to be seen promptly despite the planned appointment system.

Although the level of home visits is falling, this reduction is less sharp in the case of children. If there are other siblings or transport problems it may be difficult to bring the child to the surgery, and parents often wrongly believe that ill children should be kept in bed or that children with respiratory tract infections or a fever should not go out in the fresh air. A home visit is valuable in educating the parents.

A general practitioner is the doctor of first contact who provides continuing care and has 24-hour responsibility for all his patients. Access should be simple. Some general practitioners dislike being interrupted by telephone calls during a consultation session, but speaking directly to an anxious parent may save time and increase confidence. Outside surgery hours telephone access should be simple. A direct call diversion which would mean the general practitioner himself answering the telephone is ideal but not always possible. Alternatives should not involve more than one step—for example, an answering machine should give a number where the doctor can be contacted, not yet another number which will refer the caller elsewhere. With the advent of radiopagers and cellular telephones no general practitioner need be out of contact with his patients.

Primary care

A rota system among group practices or singlehanded family doctors, in which the doctors share their out-of-hours work with colleagues, is the ideal method of sharing night duty. Deputising services provide doctors who are not aware of the family's background, do not have access to the medical records, and are not known to the family. The doctor who sees the child may have had no training in paediatrics or in general practice, and long delays may occur. At present about a third of general practitioners use deputising services. Doctors working in these services should have adequate experience of general practice and acute illness in children, and it is hoped that the new deputising subcommittee will ensure this occurs and continues.

Preventive service

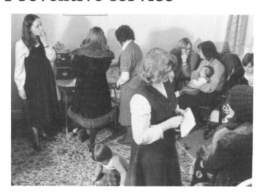

Age	Clinic activity
Birth	Home visit by GP
6 weeks	Screening check
3 months	1st immunisation DTP+Polio
5 months	2nd immunisation DTP+Polio
9 months	3rd immunisation DTP+Polio
7–10 months	1st hearing test+screening check
14 months	Screening check+measles immunisation
2½ years	Screening check
4½ years	Preschool check+DT+polio immunisation

New entrants to general practice spend a year as trainees in general practice and two years in various hospital posts, which usually include six months in paediatrics. Some experience in the community services is essential, and ideally this would be in addition to the hospital paediatric post.

Not more than one in 10 general practitioners have clinics for the regular surveillance of infants. If a general practitioner is to run his own clinics an attached health visitor is essential. Antenatal care by the family doctor prepares the family for an unrequested home visit after the mother's discharge from the maternity unit. He can then observe for himself the conditions of the family and attitudes that will mould the child's life.

During the first few months of life mothers will readily attend an efficient, welcoming baby and toddlers clinic. The baby can be weighed, a growth chart maintained, and simple advice given which will resolve many problems. The clinic also provides an opportunity for the mother to meet other mothers and discuss mutual pleasures and problems. If she finds this clinic satisfying she will continue attending so that a full programme of immunisation can be carried out. All mothers are eager to know whether their infants have normal hearing, sight, and development, and they are more ready to accept preventive health care such as immunisation from a doctor who is known to the family. Developmental screening examinations should be performed only if the general practitioner has a special interest and training in this subject. If this aspect of paediatric care is to increase vocational training schemes should allow time for the necessary skills to be acquired. Clinical medical officers in the community health service could provide these preventive services in the premises of general practitioners.

When abnormalities are detected—for example, squints, hearing disorders, speech disorders, and varying degrees of delayed development—prompt referral to the appropriate specialist is necessary.

The Royal College of General Practitioners has developed a package providing a handbook and record cards for general practitioners who wish to start preschool surveillance.

Equipment

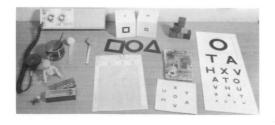

Sutures and dressings to deal with minor injuries should be available because there is often a long wait in local accident and emergency departments and management by the general practitioner is more appropriate. Equipment for resuscitating the newborn and for performing developmental screening should be available, as should equipment for examining children. Toys and other items to help the doctor talk to the child are useful. A simple screening audiometer for assessing hearing loss in children with resolving otitis is invaluable.

Primary health care team

General practitioner
Nurse
Health visitor
Midwife
Practice manager
Secretary/receptionist
(Social worker)

The primary health care team consists of the general practitioner, nurse, health visitor, and midwife, with the practice manager, receptionists, and secretary. An attached social worker is an essential part of many teams. The team meets regularly to co-ordinate and improve care. The lack of social workers in many primary health care teams reduces their effectiveness.

The health visitor provides the mother with advice on child care in the home and the clinic, and she is one of the most effective sources of health education. She also has the opportunity to teach the mother how to look after a sick child in the home. As part of the team she can feed back to the general practitioner and social worker any early warning signs of child abuse.

Communication

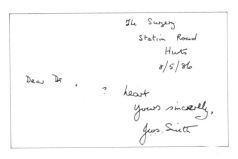

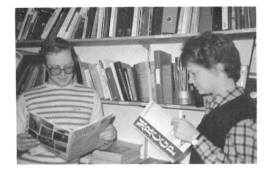

The general practitioner's letter of referral to a paediatrician should contain the following information:

• Date of birth; address.
• Family history where relevant.
• Social circumstances and details of other agencies involved.
• History and developmental history.
• History of present complaint.
• Current and previously tried medication; drug allergies.
• The reason for referral.

The consultant's reply should contain the following information:

• Extra pieces of vital information which he may have obtained.
• His own diagnosis and treatment plan.
• What he has told the family.
• When he intends to review the case.
• If he is not reviewing the case under what circumstances he wishes to see the child again.

Continuing education

The local postgraduate tutor should arrange meetings in the form of seminars so that general practitioners, clinical medical officers, and consultants can share their views and experiences.

It is becoming increasingly common for doctors to meet in small, locally based groups to discuss various topics.

Many practices are auditing the care that they are giving children in various fields such as immunisation, asthma, and upper respiratory tract infections. This trend is increasing.

Practices should have an adequate reference library with up-to-date journals and textbooks relevant to paediatric care.

SERVICES FOR CHILDREN: THE COMMUNITY

Primary and secondary care services

Primary care services for children are provided by the community health staff of the district health authority and by general practitioners and their teams. Historically, the preventive aspects of child health (surveillance, immunisation, and health education) have been the responsibility of the health authority (and, before 1974, the local authority), but increasingly general practitioners with attached health visitors are taking on this role. Integration of these primary health services is a logical development. It can be achieved in a number of ways: by organising suitable training sessions for general practitioners (and GP vocational trainees); by employing general practitioners to work as clinical medical officers to see child patients in health authority clinics; or by clinical medical officers working in general practitioners' premises.

Initially, secondary care services were mainly hospital based, but in enlightened districts consultants or their equivalents now spend more time working in the community. Clinical medical officers, as well as general practitioners, frequently act as clinical assistants to hospital paediatricians.

Computers in community child health

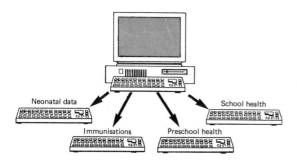

Neonatal data   School health

Immunisations   Preschool health

Many districts are using the national child health computer system, with the option of four modules: a child register with neonatal data, immunisations, and preschool health and school health modules. Basic health data are stored and distributed to general practitioners and clinic staff and appointments are sent directly for preschool health checks and immunisations. Lists of schoolchildren due for various screening tests are produced and management advice sent to the teachers.

Child health and development

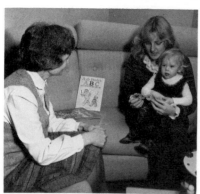

Health visitors, who are state registered nurses with additional obstetric and specific training, are based in clinics and general practitioners' surgeries. Their main role is in the home, and through health education they promote good child rearing practices. They support mothers with management problems and they are frequently responsible for some development checks. Clinical medical officers and general practitioners also carry out screening tests, but they are increasingly concerned in selective development assessment sessions.

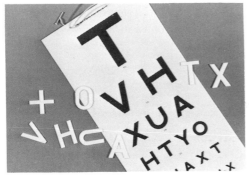

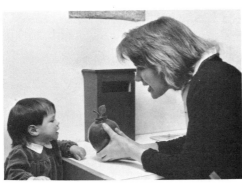

Screening—The schedules and contents of screening programmes vary enormously and few have been evaluated. The following programme recommended in the Court Report is frequently used:

Age	Main objectives and assessment
6–8 weeks	Discuss feeding problems and immunisation Exclude congenital abnormalities, e.g. congenital dislocation of the hips, cataracts Carry out simple neurodevelopmental check
8–9 months	Carry out distraction hearing tests Ensure sitting unsupported Assess manipulation Assess vision and test for squint
18 months	Ensure walking well Assess language and hearing Assess fine motor skills
3 years	Assess letter matching; carry out vision test using Snellen charts Carry out word discrimination hearing test Assess speech and language Assess fine motor and performance skills

Indices of growth, including head circumference, should be regularly plotted on a centile chart.

Hearing problems

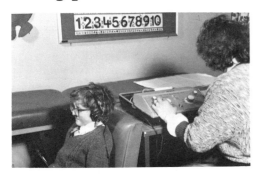

Children who fail screening tests of hearing are seen in audiology clinics staffed by an experienced community paediatrician and audiometrician. If deafness is suspected the child is referred to a consultant otologist. A child of school age, who can cooperate with audiometry, may be referred to a local clinic solely for an audiogram.

A child with severe hearing impairment requiring education at a partially hearing unit is monitored in school by the team and by a teacher of the deaf.

Immunisations

Is the baby unwell in any way?	YES/NO
Has the baby had any side effects from previous immunisation?	YES/NO
Did the baby behave normally during the first week of life?	YES/NO
Has the baby, or anyone in the immediate family, ever had fits or convulsions?	YES/NO
Is the baby developing normally?	YES/NO

Mothers can fill out a card in the waiting room at each visit for immunisation.

Immunisations should be given by a specially trained nurse who either is experienced in resuscitation techniques or has medical support nearby. The schedule recommended by the DHSS is as follows:

Age	Immunisation
13 weeks	1st diphtheria, tetanus, pertussis, polio
19–21 weeks	2nd diphtheria, tetanus, pertussis, polio
36–40 weeks	3rd diphtheria, tetanus, pertussis, polio
12–18 months	Measles
$4\frac{1}{2}$ years	Booster diphtheria, tetanus, polio
Newborn (of Afro-Asian origin only)	BCG
10–13 years	Rubella (girls only)
13 years	BCG
13–15 years	Polio, tetanus

Community care

School health

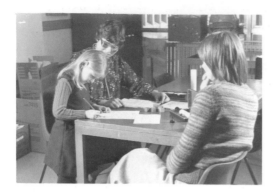

The school health team should consist of a doctor and nurse trained in educational medicine, a health visitor, and dental staff. Audiometric screening is carried out by the nurse or a technician, who may also do impedance tests to exclude serious otitis media. In some districts general practitioners have taken on the role of school doctor, and if the nurse has received appropriate training she may take over the main responsibility for screening. She checks the child's vision, height, and weight regularly, plotting the measurements on the centile chart. She may also screen for scoliosis and other medical conditions.

It is generally agreed that all children should be seen by the doctor and nurse around school entry. If this is delayed until the second term in school a questionnaire completed by the teacher can be of value. In the middle and high schools the doctor is more profitably employed reviewing only those children selected by nurse surveillance, together with information from teachers' and parents' questionnaires, or those with known special needs.

Secondary care: children with special needs

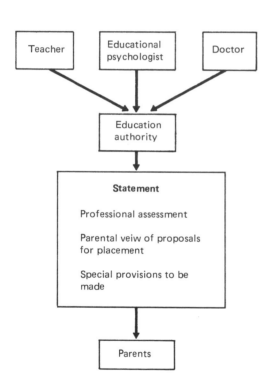

Child development centre—The team of professionals which assesses, treats, and supports the handicapped child and his family is ideally based in a district centre situated in the community or the hospital. The same integrated team will also support the child at home and in any group, unit, or school he attends.

Education Act 1981—This Act incorporates many of the recommendations of the Warnock Committee report (1978) on the special educational needs of children. Approximately 20% of the population have such requirements, and if they cannot be met by the resources and facilities of normal schools a statutory assessment and statement of needs must be made.

Parents can request this assessment whatever the age of the child; their consent is required only if the child is under 2 years of age. The assessment is frequently initiated by a professional. Assessment is carried out by the teacher, an educational psychologist, and a doctor, who is frequently the school doctor (although occasionally a consultant). The medical report will include all specialist opinions and the paramedical reports. A health authority has a duty to inform the education authority about a child who it believes may have special educational needs. The statement issued to the parents by the local education authority contains the parental view of proposals for placement and the professional assessment reports, and it lists the special provision to be made by the local health authority and district health authority. As a result of the 1981 Act special education is available, though not compulsory, for children from 2 years of age.

In the spirit of Warnock, the handicapped child should be integrated into a normal school whenever the necessary resources are available. The situation is reviewed annually and reassessment carried out at 13–14 years.

Special community clinics—Each district offers a variable service. There is scope for clinics in general and speciality paediatrics, psychiatry, ophthalmology, audiology, dietetics, enuresis, and the treatment of speech and language disorders. A special secondary immunisation clinic for complex problems, run by an experienced paediatrician, will increase the immunisation uptake rate.

Social paediatrics—Consultant paediatricians and senior clinical medical officers advise on child abuse, fostering and adoption, and children in day nurseries and in care. Together with the primary care team, they support families after a cot death or death from other causes.

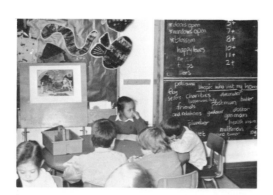

Doctors in the child health services

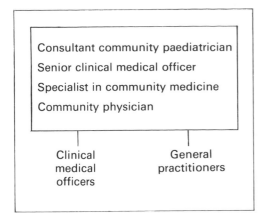

Consultant community paediatrician
Senior clinical medical officer
Specialist in community medicine
Community physician

Clinical medical officers

General practitioners

The medical team leader may be one of a number of doctors; a consultant community paediatrician or a senior clinical medical officer and, occasionally, a specialist in community medicine have the necessary clinical paediatric skills to fulfil this role. In other districts the district medical officer or a similar community physician is in charge. Community paediatricians and a number of senior clinical medical officers are fully accredited in paediatrics, with both hospital and community experience. Many other senior clinical medical officers and a few specialists in community medicine have many years' clinical experience, whereas community physicians and the newer specialists in community medicine have an epidemiological training.

Many clinical medical officers receive in-service training and they have some paediatric experience, but this is not obligatory. It is hoped that in the future they will have a three-year vocational training which will also be acceptable for general practice.

SERVICES FOR CHILDREN: OUTPATIENT CLINICS AND DAY CARE

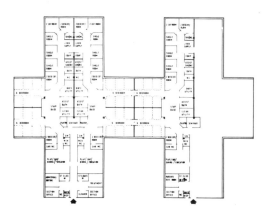

DHSS nucleus hospitals key plan: children's nursing sections

If children are to receive appropriate health care they need a spectrum of connected services: primary care from general practice and the community health service and secondary care mainly through the hospital. The hospital provides accident and emergency, outpatient, day, and inpatient services. To use resources most efficiently the district services for acutely ill children should be centralised in one department in the main hospital; ideally facilities for inpatient, outpatient, and day care should be close together.

Outpatient consultation

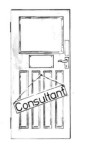 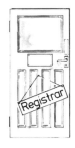 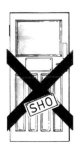

An average-sized unit cannot manage more than about 1000 new outpatients and 5000 return visits a year. Ideally all children should be seen within a week of referral, but in many units urgent cases are seen within a week and others in two or three weeks. The referral letter should describe the doctor's worries, current medication, investigations performed, and the family or social background. Referral letters are read by the consultant, who determines the date of the appointment according to the probable diagnosis. If the letter is illegible or vital information is missing a dangerous delay may occur before the child is seen. Packing the clinic with spuriously urgent cases may prevent any child from having an adequate consultation.

New patients are usually seen by a consultant or by a registrar who discusses the children with the consultant. Parents need to know that not every child can see the consultant, or fewer patients would be seen. Most parents prefer to see the same doctor each time. Considerable paediatric experience is needed before outpatient care can be provided competently and ideally a doctor with less than a year's experience in paediatrics should not do this work alone.

Indications for referral

? Diagnosis

Special expertise

Chronic disease

Special investigations

Second opinion

Families may pressurise a family doctor to seek a second opinion even though he does not consider it necessary. Most family doctors will anticipate the parents' feelings and arrange a consultation at a suitable stage. There is usually no hesitation in referring children when the diagnosis is obscure, a particular consultant has special expertise in that problem, the disease is likely to cause long-term handicap, special investigations are necessary, or the advice of a large team is appropriate. The decision is harder when the consultant is unlikely to be able to provide additional treatment but the parents may be helped to accept their doctor's explanation and management after being seen in hospital. For example, the parents of a child with recurrent upper respiratory infections may imagine that he has a serious disease and be reassured by an independent opinion.

Type of problems seen

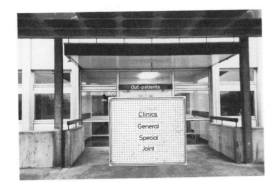

The commonest problems in new patients include recurrent respiratory tract infections, bronchial asthma, behaviour problems, enuresis, failure to thrive, recurrent abdominal pain, and convulsions. Children with systolic murmurs are referred after the murmur has been detected at routine examinations, and children with suspected urinary tract infections are often sent for further investigations.

Some chronic conditions are followed up in hospital clinics because their management demands special skill. Joint clinics may be held with specialists in diabetes, leukaemia, orthopaedics, or plastic surgery, and there may be special clinics for cystic fibrosis, gastroenterology, fits, or chronic handicaps. Children with severe asthma tend to be seen in general paediatric clinics since they form the largest single group of children with a recurring or persisting disability.

Inappropriate referrals

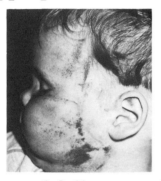

Children with suspected diabets mellitus or with features suggesting non-accidental injury should be admitted immediately; in these circumstances an outpatient referral is dangerous. Similarly children with an acute illness of unknown cause may well have recovered by the time of the appointment.

Neonatal follow-up clinics

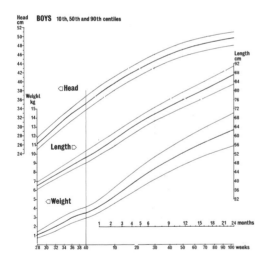

Most special care baby units arrange to follow up selected patients until they are 18 months or 2 years old. Most were born weighing under 2000 g and a few have had birth asphyxia or less common problems such as neonatal convulsions. These infants are usually seen at a separate clinic, where enough time is available for developmental assessment.

Appointment systems and accommodation

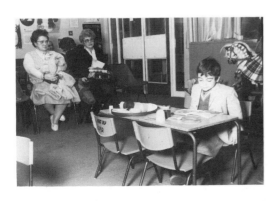

There are several problems with appointment systems: ensuring that new patients are given enough time for their consultation and that there is an allowance for patients who arrive late or default or for those with complex problems that take a long time to deal with. Children become irritable and hungry if they have to wait too long and their mothers may forget their main problems when they finally enter the consulting room.

The outpatient department for children should be designed especially for them, but in most hospitals it still has to be shared with other specialties. There should at least be a separate waiting area with furniture of the appropriate size and no stairs, lifts, or heavy doors, which could cause accidents. Rooms are needed for measuring, changing, breast-feeding, and urine collection, and the consulting room needs a small table and chair for a toddler, toys and books, and pictures on the walls and ceiling.

Outpatient clinics and day care

Communication

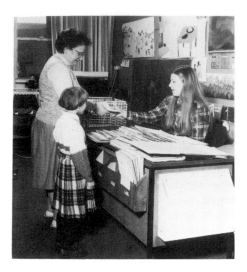

A letter sent promptly to the family doctor should contain the probable diagnosis, prognosis, and management. The history and physical findings should be noted briefly. The results of investigations can be included in a second letter to the family doctor and in another to the parents.

An efficient receptionist is the pivot of the clinic. She should like children and have sympathy with their mothers. She will be the first person to meet the family when they arrive and her kindness will affect their feelings about the unit. A paediatric nurse measures and weighs the children and collects urine specimens. In most cases the doctor can examine the child with only the mother present and no nurse.

Indications for day care

Investigations
Grommets
Hernia
Circumcision
Sigmoidoscopy

Investigations
Urine collection:
Bag
Suprapubic puncture
Catheter
Blood test
Sweat test
Sugar tolerance test
IVP
Micturating cystourethrogram

Treatment
Surgical
General
Dental
Acute attack of asthma
Chemotherapy for leukaemia
Blood transfusion

Day care is the best method of providing certain services, and though the cost needs to be considered it should not be the main reason for advocating day care. Day patients are those who attend for observation, investigation, surgery, or other treatment and who need some form of supervision, or period of recovery. The child is not separated from his parents, he sleeps at home at night, and the life of the family is less disrupted than during admission. Parents will usually prefer to bring their children to a day centre, if necessary more than once, than have them admitted. In some busy departments day care may be the only way of ensuring that there are enough beds and nurses for all the children for whom family doctors request admission.

About a third of all elective general surgery in children can be carried out in a day unit. Suitable surgical problems include aspiration of the middle ear and grommet insertion, hernia operations, circumcision, and sigmoidoscopy. There is also a place for preventive and restorative dental care, particularly in physically and mentally handicapped children. If the mother has satisfactory postoperative analgesics to give her child at home, these procedures are as safe in a day unit as in an inpatient ward. Postoperative visits or phone calls to the home by doctors or nurses are rarely necessary. The anaesthetic given must be suitable for day care, and the surgery should not be delegated to a junior doctor.

Indications for medical day care are less well defined, and the patients being seen need to be reviewed regularly to avoid overwhelming the service. The main indications are investigations, treatment of specific problems such as a severe attack of bronchial asthma or repeated chemotherapy for leukaemia, and referral from the family doctor for an opinion on admission. Children with failure to thrive or developmental delay, who were previously admitted for long periods, can be investigated completely in a day care unit.

Day care can complement an outpatient visit, especially with necessary but difficult investigations. Taking blood for measuring anticonvulsant concentrations from a kicking, fat toddler can be an ordeal for everyone in a hectic outpatient clinic; in the day care unit it may be much easier. Some tests, such as sweat tests or sugar tolerance tests, take a long time but the day care unit's playroom reduces the ordeal. Toddlers are often distressed by an intravenous pyelogram and even more by a micturating cystogram, but preliminary sedation in the day care unit and a bed to sleep in afterwards may reduce the anxiety and discomfort.

Walk-in day cases

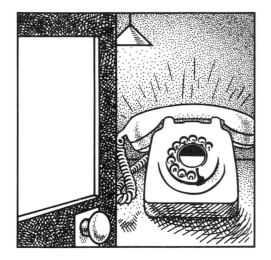

Family doctors may be encouraged to refer particular groups of patients to the unit on a "phone and walk in" basis. These may include patients with suspected urinary tract infections, where a properly collected specimen is crucial, or those with bronchial asthma, in whom early treatment may abort an acute attack. Pressure from parents may persuade a family doctor to send a child to the unit rather than wait for an outpatient appointment. This is an abuse of the system and will not lead to the satisfactory management of a child with a chronic problem.

Some paediatric units in inner city areas have taken this idea a stage further and provided an open clinic for a few hours each day where family doctors can send patients without appointment for a second opinion. Among other advantages, such a clinic may prevent children being brought to the accident and emergency department at any time of the day or night and seeing a doctor who has not had paediatric experience. These clinics must be managed by doctors with considerable experience and avoid becoming another way of fragmenting primary care.

Staffing and accommodation

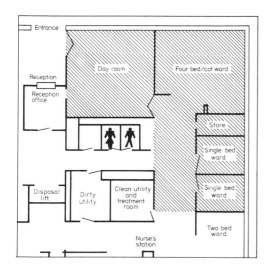

A senior house officer supervised by a registrar can be responsible for a day unit on a part-time basis; and it is also particularly suitable for part-time paediatric nurses. Both the staff and the accommodation need to be separated from those of the inpatient unit, since the pace and type of work are different and cannot be mixed without loss of efficiency.

In district hospitals the day care unit for children can be a four-bedded ward separated from the main unit by doors. There are many advantages in having an operating theatre nearby. Ideally there should be a quiet area, a section for procedures, and a play area, where observation is easy but sound is not readily transmitted.

SERVICES FOR CHILDREN: ACCIDENT AND EMERGENCY DEPARTMENTS AND INPATIENTS

Accident and emergency departments

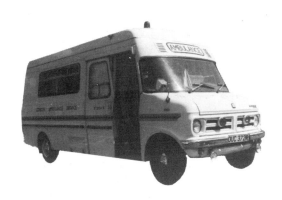

Accidents and emergencies in children are usually managed in the main department, where about three-quarters of the patients are adults and where few of the nursing and medical staff have any postgraduate paediatric training. In most hospitals a member of the paediatric team is on call to give a second opinion to the accident and emergency officer. Equipment of appropriate size for varying ages can only easily be available if a resuscitation room is equipped specifically for children. A separate waiting room, consulting room, and drug cupboard may also reduce many of the disadvantages of children being seen in a mainly adult department.

In many inner city areas the accident and emergency department provides a great deal of primary care, particularly at evenings and weekends. If the paediatric senior house officer on call spends most of his time giving primary care he may find it difficult to fulfil his other commitments, which may include resuscitation of the newborn, management of infants on ventilators, and care of severely ill children.

Admission to hospital

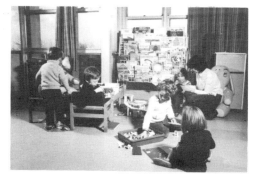

Although it has long been DHSS policy that children should be admitted only to children's wards, this has not been implemented in many hospitals, partly because of the persistence of specialised units for ear, nose, and throat surgery and ophthalmology, where children and adults are nursed in the same ward. Children need nurses and ancillary staff attuned to their needs to prevent unnecessary distress. Although the admission of a mother with the child may reduce this trauma some mothers are daunted by the unwelcoming attitudes of staff and primitive accommodation.

Indications for admission

Surgery
Urgent investigations
Nursing
Complex problems

The severely ill child clearly needs to be admitted. Children with problems needing admission include those with fractures requiring operation or traction and those with suspected acute appendicitis. Some children need urgent medical investigations—for example, a lumbar puncture—and others have urgent social and medical reasons such as non-accidental injuries. Some medical patients need nursing and treatment that cannot be provided at home, such as intravenous treatment for bronchial asthma or oxygen and tube feeding for bronchiolitis. Complex problems may need the opinions of several specialists, who may be better coordinated by a short admission, though most investigations can now be performed in a day care unit. Severely ill children needing intensive monitoring or ventilation are usually nursed on the intensive care unit, managed jointly by the paediatrician and anaesthetist in charge of the unit.

Admission procedure

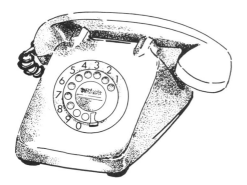

When direct admission is sought the family doctor usually discusses the problem with the paediatric senior house officer. This telephone conversation helps to clarify the problem and decide whether there are any special social reasons contributing to the admission. Arrangements can also be discussed for a possible early discharge or ways of avoiding admission. The average length of stay for paediatric inpatients is three to four days but if beds are to be available for every admission requested the average occupancy cannot exceed 70%. This means that during epidemics patients may have to be discharged sooner than usual and followed up in the day care unit or outpatient clinic.

Common reasons for admission

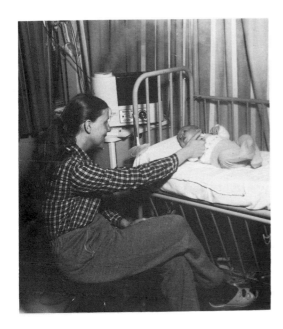

The sudden deterioration that may occur in infants with bronchiolitis or severe asthma has encouraged family doctors to send these patients into hospital. Some of these children could be nursed at home if the family doctor visited them often enough to admit them if they deteriorated. But general practitioners are under pressure from parents to admit children to hospital. Such expectations are hard to resist if there are beds available, and children may be admitted for a short period during the acute phase of the illness. Children with a first febrile convulsion are usually admitted to exclude meningitis and to allay the parents' fears.

The introduction of effective prophylactic drugs appears to have persuaded parents that they do not have to wait a week or so for the natural history of an asthmatic attack to take place. Many units now have an open-house system so that a child with a severe attack can be seen in the day care unit and be admitted if his attack is not quickly relieved. This early treatment may result in more children being admitted, but they have symptoms for a shorter period and miss less school. Repeated admissions also indicate that the management is ineffective and needs to be changed. Most medical investigations can now be carried out in a day care unit, and about a third of the paediatric surgery at present performed in the inpatient ward could be carried out in a day care unit.

Nurses in paediatric wards

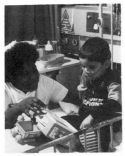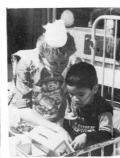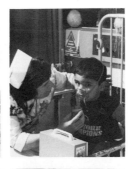
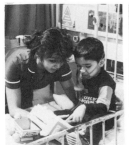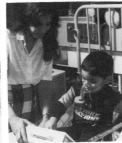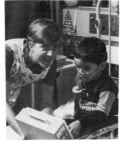

The shift system results in each child being nursed by six to eight different nurses each week, despite the fact that each nurse may look after the same group of children each time she is on duty. The mother is therefore the only person who can provide continuity of care for a child, and the admission of the child without the mother is likely to aggravate any feeding or behaviour problems.

Mothers

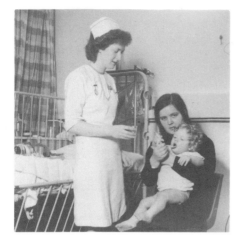

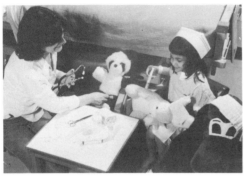

The attitudes of staff towards mothers determine whether the mothers want to stay. The ward sister will set an example and show that they are complementary to the nurses and not usurping the nurses' role. The resident mother needs basic comforts including a folding bed, a cupboard for her clothes, a bathroom, and a room where she can chat to other mothers. She needs to know where to find linen, make tea, and obtain a meal. A list of guidelines will give her more confidence. Some prefer to go home for short periods, especially in the evenings, and they should be encouraged to do so. If a mother does not want to stay in the unit she should not be pressed. Normal siblings can stay with the patient and mother. More than half of mothers will stay with their children if they are given the opportunity and this should not be related to the child's age. Some anaesthetists allow the mother to go with the child to the anaesthetic room.

In the ward the mother can carry out the usual care, including feeding, changing, and bathing. She can also take the child for investigations and can keep fluid charts, collect urine, and in some cases observe the flow of intravenous fluids. Selected mothers can be taught simple nursing procedures such as temperature recording and tube feeding. During admission the mother learns more about nursing a sick child and gains confidence. The nurses can assess the mother's competence in managing the child and her attitude towards him and find it easier to assess the appropriate time for discharge. Student nurses may learn a great deal from an experienced mother about the skilled and sensitive care of a young child.

Play is a child's work, not simply amusement. A skilled play leader can help the child to play out the events of the admission by allowing him to handle syringes and the other equipment and she can discover with the mother how the child feels. Most wards have a part-time or full-time schoolteacher.

Staff strain

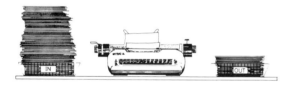

If the admission policy is working well most of the children on the ward are acutely ill. Many are discharged shortly after they begin to improve so the wards no longer have convalescent patients. The short period of admission and the high discharge rate for each bed produce continuous emotional strains on nursing, junior medical staff, and secretarial staff. The high rate of admissions is similar to that in an intensive care unit, but the allocation of nurses does not usually take this into account. Staff morale and quality of care can easily fall when nursing and medical staff are working continuously under high pressure. Many units do not have the funds to bring the nursing establishment up to an adequate level and others would find it difficult to recruit enough nurses even if funds were available. Providing more day care is often the only solution compatible with providing a continuous service to the child community.

Infectious diseases

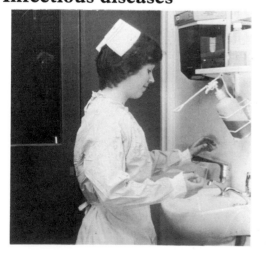

The most common infectious disease requiring admission is acute gastroenteritis. Most children with acute gastroenteritis can be managed at home, but those requiring intravenous fluids or those with poor social conditions may need admission. Ideally these children should be nursed in an annexe to the children's ward. Properly designed cubicles with double doors allow barrier nursing and help to prevent cross-infection. Unless the mother is admitted with the child emotional and social isolation is an inevitable consequence of the physical isolation. Social and emotional problems present before admission may be increased by admitting these children to an adult infectious diseases unit because paediatric nurses are essential. Children with measles, chickenpox, mumps, or scarlet fever rarely need to be admitted, although they may be severely ill for a short part of the disease. Children with heavily infected eczema and those with leukaemia who have developed chickenpox are best managed in a barrier-nursed cubicle on a children's ward.

Preparation for admission to the paediatric unit

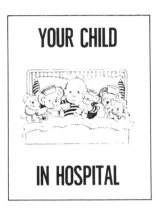

An admission booklet prepares the mother and child for what they can expect in the ward. Several of these booklets are specially prepared with children in mind and include pictures which they can colour in before arrival. For planned admissions the child can be shown round the ward after finishing the outpatient consultation. As a large proportion of the child population will be admitted or seen at hospital at some stage a few schools arrange trips to the local hospital. There are now several excellent books written for children about hospital and the mother can inform herself about ward life as she reads about it to the child.

The newborn

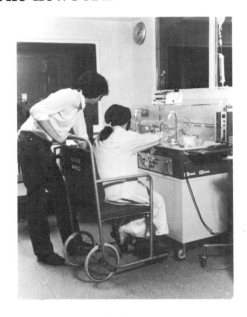

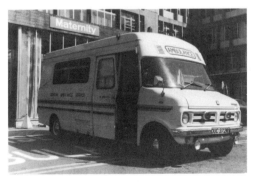

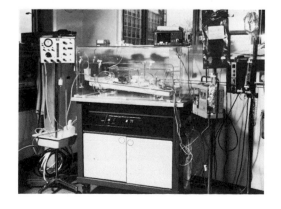

The largest number of infants in hospital are newborn infants, who may account for 3000 admissions a year, compared with 2000 in the paediatric wards. Most of these babies are completely well and in many units they stay next to their mothers throughout the 24 hours. The length of stay depends on the policy of the unit. During his stay the infant should be examined at least once by a member of the paediatric staff and in some units will also be examined by the obstetric junior staff. The mother is taught to care for her infant mainly by the midwife in the antenatal and neonatal period. Some wards also have nursery nurses.

About 15% of newborn infants need special nursing care. Most of these infants weigh less than 2000 g at birth, are preterm, have had perinatal asphyxia, or have respiratory problems. Some have feeding difficulties or need phototherapy. To avoid separating all these infants from their mothers some units have provided an "intermediate" ward, which is a postnatal ward with nurses who can provide simple forms of neonatal special care. This can reduce the number of infants going to the intensive neonatal care unit from 15% to 7%.

A new mother may be frightened and bewildered by the complicated equipment and the appearance of the baby; she may be helped by a preliminary explanation by a member of the medical or nursing staff before she enters the unit. This explanation can be amplified by a pamphlet. If nursing staff welcome the mother she will not be afraid to visit the unit frequently to touch, change, feed, and later breast-feed her infant. Brothers and sisters should visit the baby from shortly after birth, and a suitable play area and toys will be needed. The social worker to the unit will offer to see the parents personally or in a group to try to reduce stress.

Some units (regional intensive care units) receive babies of extremely low birth weight and those needing artificial ventilation. An increasing number of mothers are transferred to these units before delivery to minimise birth asphyxia and avoid transporting a sick infant. Separation of a mother from her family may be unavoidable and visiting difficult because of the distance and cost.

Nurses may find it stressful to work in such a unit, especially at night, when staff shortages are common. The design of units with large windows so that the staff can see the sunrise, trees, and birds may reduce this feeling of isolation, although it may make it more difficult to maintain constant temperature.

The special care unit often has a separate establishment of nurses who do not work in any other part of the hospital. In Britain most consultant paediatricians divide their time between the care of newborn and older children. The registrar may have special responsibilities for the newborn during the day but is often on call for the whole department at night. Senior houses officers are often responsible for both the newborn and older children at night but mainly for one or the other during the day.

CHILD ABUSE

100 deaths

Sexual abuse:
1 in 10 girls
1 in 15 boys

In Britain as many as a hundred children may die each year from inflicted injuries. Before the age of 16 years at least one in ten girls and one in fifteen boys will have been sexually assaulted. The peak incidence of the first sexual assault is about the age of 8 years, although disclosure by the child is later—usually in early adolesence. About 80% of the children are sexually abused by persons known to them, often a father, stepfather, male relation, or co-habitee of the mother. A borough of about a quarter of a million population can expect 500 new cases of sexual abuse a year but probably only one in five of them will come forward.

Definitions

Physical injury

Neglect

Emotional neglect

Sexual abuse

Potential abuse

A parent or another supervisor can harm a child by a deliberate act or failure to provide adequate care. The types of abuse have been divided into the following groups:
(a) *Physical injury*, which may have been inflicted deliberately or by failure to provide a safe environment.
(b) *Neglect* in providing food and warmth may impair physical health and development.
(c) *Emotional neglect* or rejection may impair normal emotional development.
(d) *Sexual abuse* (see page 113).
(e) There may be a high risk of *potential abuse* where another child in the household has been harmed or a large number of risk factors are present.

Recognition

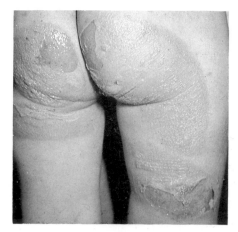

Child abuse should be suspected, especially in a child aged under 3 years, if any of the following features are present:
• There has been delay between an injury occurring and the parent seeking medical help.
• The explanation of the injury is inadequate, discrepant, or too plausible.
• The child or sibling has a history of non-accidental or suspicious injury.
• There is evidence of earlier injury.
• The child has often been brought to the family doctor or accident department for little apparent reason.
• The parents show disturbed behaviour or unusual reactions to the child's injuries or have a history of psychiatric illness.
• The child shows obvious neglect or failure to thrive.

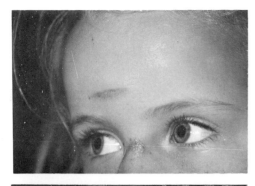

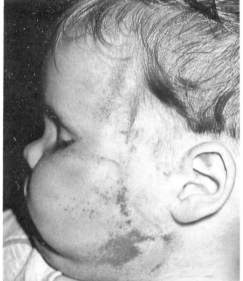

Injuries may be similar to those encountered after a genuine accident, but certain injuries are typical of abuse:
• Burns, abrasions, or small bruises on the face.
• Injuries to the mouth or torn frenulum of the lip.
• Finger-shaped bruises.
• Subconjunctival or retinal haemorrhages.
• Bruises of different ages.

If non-accidental injury is suspected the child should be undressed completely, examined fully, and careful notes made of all findings using drawings. If suspicions are not allayed the child should be admitted immediately to hospital under the care of a consultant paediatrician. If possible the suspicions should not be communicated to the parents at this stage as they may refuse to allow admission.

If the parents refuse to agree to the child being admitted or want to remove him from hospital too soon the social services department may seek a Place of Safety Order, which allows a child to be kept in hospital for 28 days. In an emergency the police can secure an immediate Place of Safety Order but this lasts only 8 days. The fact that children with genuinely accidental injuries will occasionally be admitted unnecessarily should not deter any doctor from admitting a child when there is reasonable doubt about the cause of an injury. Within a few days a case conference is convened to try to determine whether an injury was accidental and whether the child should be allowed home, taken into care voluntarily, or taken into care through court proceedings (see chapter on social services).

Sexual abuse

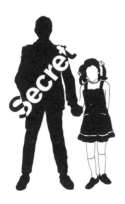

Sexual abuse is the involvement of dependent, developmentally immature children and adolescents in sexual activities they do not truly comprehend, to which they are unable to give informed consent, and which violate the social taboos of family roles or are against the law. In the past few years the number of cases identified has increased as the public has become more aware of the problem and professional staff have become more skilled at recognising sexual abuse. A child's statement that he or she is being abused should be accepted as true until proved otherwise. Children rarely lie about sexual abuse. False allegations are, in any event, a sign of a disturbed family environment and an indication that a child may need help.

Presentation

Injuries to genitalia or anus

Recurrent urinary infection

Sexual explicitness

Sudden changes in behaviour

Sexual abuse presents in three main ways:
    allegations by the child or an adult;
    injuries to the genitalia or anus;
    suspicious features.

Suspicious features include unexplained recurrent urinary tract infections, or sexual explicitness in play, drawing, language, or behaviour. There may be sudden or unexplained changes in behaviour—for example, sleep disturbance with nightmares, fear of men, or loss of trust in those near them. Self-destructive behaviour may occur, including the taking of overdoses of drugs or running away from home. Most of these physical or behavioural signs have other explanations and should do no more than raise the possibility of child sexual abuse for professionals puzzled by a child's behaviour.

Child abuse

Investigation

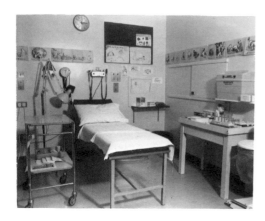

Quick, highly co-ordinated work by doctors, social workers, and the police is required and they may meet informally to plan the investigations. If the abuse has occurred within the previous 48 hours the investigation may need to include the collection of forensic evidence by a suitably qualified doctor. The child should not be subjected to repeated medical examinations but referred initially to a suitably experienced doctor who is sensitive to the needs of children and the issues involved and who is experienced at giving medical evidence in court. This doctor could be a paediatrician, police surgeon, or other doctor. Social workers, police, and doctors should not subject the child to unnecessary repeated interviewing. The medical examination should be conducted in a suitable clinical setting in the paediatric department of the local hospital.

The first formal case conference involving other agencies is likely to be called only when the outcome of the investigation is known and further assessment and planning are needed. Admission to hospital allows the initial investigations to be carried out, as well as providing a place of safety until the risks can be assessed at the formal case conference. Initial management should provide care for acute medical, emotional, and social problems, ensure that the abuse stops, and encourage the formulation of plans for treatment while complying with legal requirements. Court sentences with a requirement to undertake treatment without a prison sentence have been effective in some cases.

Sexual abuse, particularly where a person known to the child was involved and where the abuse continued over a long period, can be followed by serious long-term effects. These include the post-traumatic syndrome, suicidal behaviour, psychiatric illness, and problems with relationships and sexual adjustment.

Long-term effects

Post traumatic

Suicidal behaviour

Psychiatric illness

Problems with relationships and sexual adjustment

Prevention

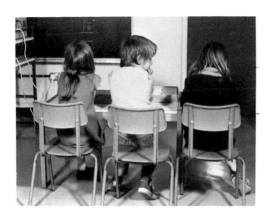

Increasing the knowledge and awareness of the public and all professionals involved with children will result in the earlier reporting of sexual abuse. Clear local guidelines on procedure and good co-operation between investigating agencies will improve the management of these very difficult problems. Voluntary organisations and self-help groups offering informal counselling through drop-in centres or telephone lines enable some children or families to seek help.

Teaching children how to protect themselves offers the greatest potential for prevention. The prime responsibility lies with the parents, but some schools have started work in this subject within the broad context of health and safety education. Some children have confided experiences to their teachers as a result of these programmes.

SERVICES FOR CHILDREN: SOCIAL SERVICES

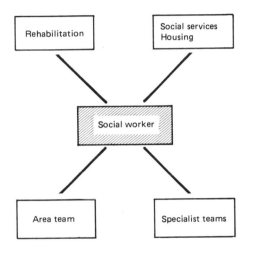

Many children seen in hospital have social as well as medical problems, and a medical social worker can help to ensure that the whole family receives appropriate care. Health visitors work closely with social workers and many share the observation and support needed by some families. The medical social worker in the paediatric department is part of the community-based service and can decide whether the social work for the family should take place in the hospital or the community. Most of her time is spent helping parents with marital problems and teaching the skills of being a parent. In paediatric units and child psychiatric clinics experienced social workers may work with particular families over a long period. Medical social workers help mothers to obtain services, especially for children with handicaps, and they link child and parents with specialist units providing temporary care, fostering, or adoption. They also supervise the rehabilitation of children who have been abused.

Child abuse

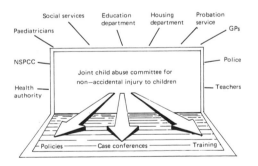

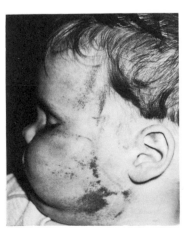

Inflicted physical injury is only one aspect of abnormal child rearing: others are emotional deprivation, physical neglect, failure to thrive, and proneness to accidents. Accurate diagnosis is essential and must be made against a background of a wide variety of normal child-rearing patterns and the vast majority of genuine childhood accidents. A joint child abuse committee for non-accidental injury coordinates the policies of various agencies, provides guidelines, arranges training to increase awareness of the problem, and reviews the work of case conferences.

If a social worker suspects non-accidental injury she checks whether the child is on the child protection register (maintained by the social services department) and whether the family is known to the social services department, the health visitor, or the National Society for the Prevention of Cruelty to Children (NSPCC). Social workers then decide whether admission to hospital should be requested or whether the child should be taken into care or left at home. Parents will usually accept admission to hospital, where the child will be cared for and helped sympathetically and confidentially. A child can be fully examined and medical, social, and psychiatric investigations started. The family doctor must be told at an early stage and nursing and medical staff should be aware of the reason for admission, although this suspicion should not be discussed with the parents at this stage.

If the parents refuse a child's admission or try to remove him too soon the consultant and hospital social worker usually ask the social services department to seek a Place of Safety Order, which allows the hospital to detain the child for 28 days.

Social services

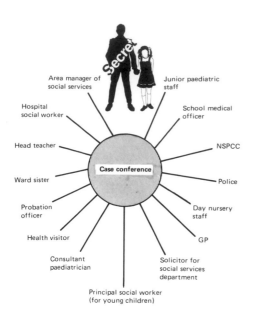

Within a few days a case conference is convened to try to determine whether an injury was accidental, to notify the register, and to decide whether the child should be allowed home, taken into care voluntarily, or removed from home through court proceedings. Psychiatric help may be offered to the family. The selected key worker (usually a social worker) sees the family regularly and the case is kept under review by the principal social worker to decide when the child may be removed from the child protection register. All the interested agencies are asked to attend subsequent conferences and for their opinion on removal from the register. After the child's name has been removed from the register the case records are destroyed. Case conferences can only recommend, and their lack of "teeth" to implement their decisions may be frustrating.

The poor long-term results of children in care make social workers reluctant to separate a child from his parents unless evidence of serious injury is conclusive. They may differ from doctors in their estimation of the degree of parental incompetence or personality disorder, but the social services department makes the final decision. If a child is removed from his parents fostering may prove more effective than placing the child in a children's home; it is also cheaper.

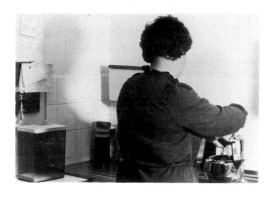

Mothers of injured infants often already have a social worker, who may find it difficult to defend the child's rights against the mother's needs. The parents may blame the social worker for their child being put on the child protection register. The appointment of a solicitor for the child does not necessarily help if he receives his brief from the mother, who may have done the injury, and he may have little experience in child care. The magistrates' court may appoint a guardian *ad litem*, who is usually an experienced independent social worker, to advise the court on action which would be in the child's best interest.

Practical preventive help—The use of social services departments' ancillary services may allow children to stay at home. Home helps are particularly helpful for single parents, especially fathers. Peripatetic foster parents may enable children to remain in their own homes. Day nurseries, nursery schools, and opportunity playgroups help reduce the stress on parents and allow the physical and emotional development of the child to be monitored. A few day nurseries have been set up to teach mothering skills; the mother's interaction with the child can be observed and encouraged and she can be taught simple domestic skills.

Professional problems

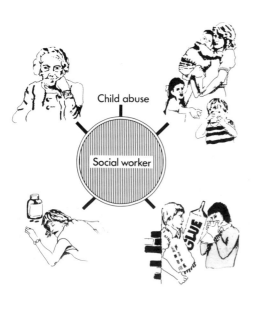

Most social workers manage problems in every age group (generic practice). The social worker looking after a family will therefore have little experience of specific paediatric problems such as child abuse or chronic handicap in infancy, as these are relatively rare. The family may have a new worker every few years, who may find it difficult to help with evolving problems in a handicapped child. Specialist social workers supervise the field workers but may not be easily available in a crisis.

The lack of precise definitions of problems and of their effects highlights the need for more research into the work of social workers. Too little attention has been paid to the feasibility of providing all the services proposed by governments, and there have been few studies into the effectiveness of social work methods. Much of the research has been by sociologists rather than social workers, which has made it difficult to translate research findings into practice. Social workers themselves need to take part in this research.

USEFUL INFORMATION

Acute herpetic gingivostomatitis

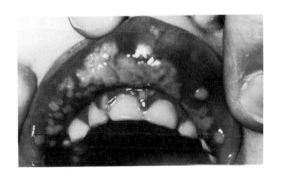

Primary infection of the mucous membranes of the mouth is the commonest infection with herpes simplex in childhood. It usually occurs at 1 to 4 years. A high fever and refusal to eat are accompanied by red swollen gums which bleed easily. There are white plaques about 3 mm in diameter or painful shallow ulcers with a red rim on the buccal mucosa, gums, tongue, and palate, and the regional lymph nodes are enlarged and tender. This is a self-limiting disease which resolves in about 10 days.

Treatment consists of keeping the mouth clean and maintaining hydration. The child might have to be admitted to hospital to prevent dehydration from refusal to drink. Regular doses of paracetamol elixir and frequent small volumes of a glucose solution or milk should be given. Fluids may cause less pain if a drinking straw is used, and jelly and ice cream may be taken easily, but citrus juices should be avoided because they increase the pain. Gentian violet solution should not be used.

Anal fissure

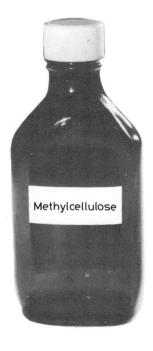

Methylcellulose

An anal fissure causes severe pain on defecation because the lesion is stretched as the stool is being passed. Fresh blood may be seen on the surface of the stool. The mucosal tear, which may occur at any point on the circumference at the mucocutaneous junction of the anus, may be visible but the lesion may be very small or too high to be seen. Fissures are usually the result of trauma to the anal margin by the passage of hard stools. This constipation may be the result of inadequate intake of fluid during a febrile illness. As a result of the pain the child resists defecation and the stools become hard and the symptoms more severe. Without treatment chronic constipation sometimes occurs with overflow diarrhoea.

The stools are kept soft by ensuring an adequate fluid intake and the addition of methylcellulose liquid (Cologel) 5 ml three times daily for a month and daily for a further month. The child then regains confidence that defecation will not be painful. It is essential that this course of treatment should be completed as a fissure takes a long time to heal. Surgical excision of the fissure or stretching of the anus is rarely needed if medical treatment is adequate.

A rectal polyp is a rarer cause of rectal bleeding, but the absence of pain helps to distinguish it from a fissure.

Useful information

Cervical lymphadenopathy (non-suppurative)

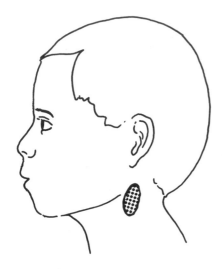

In children aged over 2 years cervical lymphadenopathy usually affects the tonsillar nodes, but more distal nodes in the neck may be affected. Viral or bacterial infection in the upper respiratory tract spreads to these lymph nodes, which change in size with each acute infection. Despite these wide changes in size the nodes seldom disappear completely for several years.

If the nodes do not change in size between two observations a month apart the possibility of tuberculosis should be considered and a tuberculin test performed.

Generalised lymphadenopathy suggests the possibility of infectious mononucleosis, leukaemia, or lymphoma. A full blood count should be performed and a blood film examined for evidence of leukaemia. If the Monospot screening test for infectious mononucleosis is negative bone marrow examination should be considered and blood should be taken for a toxoplasma dye test and cytomegalovirus antibody titre. If all these tests are negative a surgeon should be consulted to consider biopsy to exclude malignant disease.

Constipation

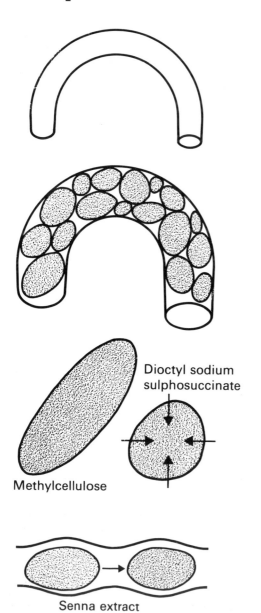

Dioctyl sodium
sulphosuccinate

Methylcellulose

Senna extract

Constipation is an alteration in bowel habit with the passage of hard stools and a reduction in the frequency of stools. Normal children may pass stools between four times a day and once every four days. Any child with an acute illness tends to eat and drink less than normal and he passes fewer stools. Apart from ensuring that fluid intake is adequate no treatment is required. If there is an inadequate intake of fluid the stools may become hard and produce an anal fissure. The pain produced during defecation by the fissure may make the child reluctant to pass stools so that he holds them back by crossing his legs. Several days may pass before the child passes a formed stool, which is then voluminous and may cause severe pain.

Colonic inertia with overflow soiling—If the child persists in refusing to pass stools chronic constipation follows. The whole colon becomes distended with firm stool and the reflex urge to defecate is lost as a result of the persistent distension of the rectum. At this stage enormous masses of faeces can be palpated through the abdominal wall and be detected on rectal examination. Liquid stool may trickle continuously around the masses and escape with gas through the anus. Parents may complain about this continual loss of fluid stool and call it diarrhoea without realising that there is underlying constipation. The doctor will not be misled if he examines the abdomen and rectum. In some children there is no obvious history of an anal fissure but bowel training has been attempted before the age of 2 years.

By the time the child is seen by a doctor the problem has often been present for several months or years and any emotional problems present may be primary or secondary to the physical problem. Most of these children can be managed by medicines, and a child psychiatrist should be consulted about those who do not improve quickly or relapse.

The cause of the problem is discussed with both parents and the child using simple diagrams, and they should be told that aperients will be needed for a prolonged period, at least for a year, otherwise relapse will occur. The following three drugs are given initially together: (a) methylcellulose liquid (Cologel) 450 mg in 5 ml three times daily, (b) dioctyl sodium sulphosuccinate (Dioctyl-Medo) 12.5 mg in 5 ml three times daily, and (c) senna extract (Senokot) 5 ml at night. The dose of senna extract is increased by 5 ml every third night until there is a daily bowel action or until the maximum dose of 15 ml is given. The first drug makes the stools soft, the second is a detergent and penetrates into the stool, and the third acts by propelling the stool. The child should be asked to sit on the lavatory at the same time each day to encourage reflex defecation. He must be seen initially each week and then at monthly intervals to ensure that the medicine is being taken. The doses of the drugs are gradually reduced after about three months and a regular habit has been regained. Relapse is common and the parents should be warned about this possibility. Suppositories and enemas and the manual removal of faeces can rarely be justified except in children with cerebral palsy.

Passing stools in unusual places such as behind curtains indicates a severe behaviour disorder, which needs referral to a child psychiatrist.

Haemoglobinopathies: normal haematological values and diagnosis

Normal ranges		
	Haemoglobin (g/dl)	Mean corpuscular volume (fl)
½–1 year	10·5–13·5	70–80
1–4 years	11·0–14·0	70–82
4–7 years	11·5–13·5	76–86
Adult	13 – 15	80–100

Mean corpuscular haemoglobin concentration is constant throughout life (30–34 g/dl)

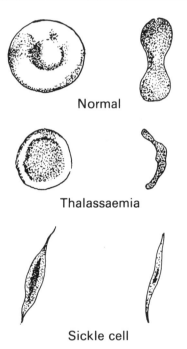

Normal

Thalassaemia

Sickle cell

Normal ranges for haemoglobin concentrations and red cell indices vary with age. The normal ranges printed on standard report forms are derived from adult studies and their use for children may result in a wrong diagnosis, especially of iron deficiency anaemia.

The child with severe anaemia due to sickle cell anaemia or thalassaemia major receives an abnormal gene from each parent, who has no symptoms.

In sickle cell anaemia there is a chronic haemolytic anaemia with superimposed crises due to local sickling, marrow aplasia, or acute haemolysis. Hypoxaemia causes deformity of the red cells with local sickling, which results in blocking of capillaries and further hypoxia and sickling. Ischaemia distal to the local sickling lesion causes bone, chest, or abdominal pain or infarcts in the brain, spleen, or kidneys. The child's parents who both have the trait (or a child with the trait) develop a sickling crisis or mild anaemia only if very severe prolonged hypoxaemia occurs. Diagnosis depends on detecting haemoglobin S alone on the haemoglobin electrophoresis of the child with sickle cell anaemia and haemoglobin S and haemoglobin A in both parents.

The most common type of thalassaemia in this country is β-thalassaemia, in which there is reduced synthesis of the β chain of globin leading to reduced synthesis of haemoglobin A and hypochromic microcytic anaemia. Synthesis of haemoglobin F and haemoglobin A_2 are not affected and so the percentages of haemoglobin F and A_2 are increased.

Two genes for thalassaemia are present in a child with thalassaemia major and one in those with thalassaemia minor. The child with thalassaemia major has severe chronic haemolytic anaemia with a very large liver and spleen and later enlargement of the frontal and malar bones due to bone marrow hyperplasia. He usually needs regular blood transfusions and desferrioxamine throughout his life. Thalassaemia minor causes mild or no anaemia. The blood picture is similar to that of iron deficiency anaemia but the mean cell volume (MCV) is disproportionately reduced compared with the red cell count (RBC) and haemoglobin levels; the ratio MCV/RBC is less than 12 and the serum iron level is normal. The diagnosis is confirmed by finding a raised percentage of haemoglobin A_2 or haemoglobin F, or both.

If thalassaemia minor or sickle cell trait is suspected during a routine antenatal clinic blood count, the father should also be tested immediately. If he has a similar abnormality the possibility that the fetus has a severe haemoglobinopathy should be considered and further expert opinion sought as a matter of urgency.

Jaundice due to hepatitis A virus

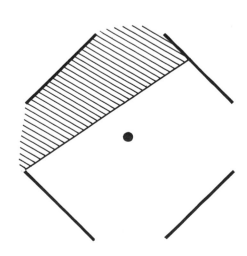

Infectious hepatitis is most commonly due to hepatitis A virus. Before jaundice appears there is often headache, anorexia, nausea, vomiting, abdominal pain, and occasionally fever. The liver may be enlarged and tender, and the spleen and lymph nodes may also be enlarged. Jaundice starts as the fever subsides, and as the jaundice increases the child's appetite improves. The urine is dark because of bile and the stools may be very pale. Jaundice lasts for 8–11 days. In children under 3 years, especially those in institutions, hepatitis may occur without jaundice.

If a child wants to stay in bed he should be allowed to, but prolonged bed rest is not essential. While there is anorexia or vomiting small volumes of glucose–electrolyte mixture flavoured with fruit juice should be given every hour during the day. As the appetite returns a normal diet may be given with no restriction of fat. No drugs are needed though some clinicians recommend vitamin supplements. Viral hepatitis is one of the mildest childhood infections and the prognosis is excellent.

The patient is potentially infectious for no more than a week after the onset of jaundice. The virus is spread by the faecal–oral route, and spread can be prevented by hand washing and by boiling food utensils for at least a minute.

When features are typical no tests are needed and the child should be nursed in his own home. Drowsiness or jaundice lasting longer than two weeks should prompt a further opinion.

Useful information

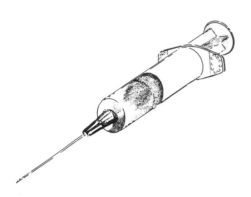

Prophylaxis—Type A viral hepatitis has an incubation period of 15–40 days with an average of 30 days. Most human sera, and therefore most human globulin preparations, contain antibody, and if this is given by injection during the incubation period it protects against the disease. The indications for giving this injection are controversial and vary between countries and units. Hepatitis A infections in children are usually mild and confer lifelong immunity, but the incidence of such infections has declined recently in northern Europe, though in southern Europe most people are infected by the time they are adults. In adults hepatitis A is more severe but rarely causes persisting or serious liver disease. In future it is more likely that adults will contract the disease from their children. Nevertheless, globulin should be used only within the incubation period, and preferably within 15 days of contact, and if there is some special reason to fear hepatitis in a sibling or adult. In future it may be thought that all parents of children with hepatitis should be protected and that only gammaglobulin preparations known to contain anti-hepatitis A antibody should be used.

In countries outside Britain where hepatitis B is common different advice on prophylaxis may be more appropriate.

Tetanus in the wounded: prevention

Give human tetanus immunoglobulin if		
Patient		*Wound*
Not immunised or immunity unknown	*and*	Over 6 h old or tissue damage or penetrating or cannot be cleaned

Surgical toilet of a wound is of prime importance since the removal of foreign bodies and dead tissue helps to prevent the growth of tetanus bacilli. The track of the wound should be opened up and all dead tissue removed. Wounds that are heavily contaminated with soil or those with severe contusion must not be sutured initially.

Active immunisation is provided by a course of adsorbed toxoid. A basic course comprises three doses—the first immediately after the injury, the second about six weeks later, and the third about 6–12 months after the second. Booster doses should be given every 10 years unless the patient has in the meantime received a dose after an injury. The importance of returning for the complete course of toxoid and booster doses must be emphasised to the patient.

If the patient has had a complete course or a booster dose of toxoid within five years no additional measures are needed for tetanus prevention. If the booster dose was given over five years earlier one dose should be given.

If the patient has not been actively immunised or his immunity is unknown and the wound is over six hours old, associated with tissue damage, or is penetrating or cannot properly be cleaned human tetanus immunoglobulin (250 units) should be given in addition to starting the course of active immunisation with toxoid. If human tetanus immunoglobulin is not available penicillin should be given for at least five days. The dose of benzylpenicillin is 200 mg/kg/24 h in divided doses by bolus injection intravenously or 50 mg/kg/24 h by intramuscular injection.

Vulvovaginitis

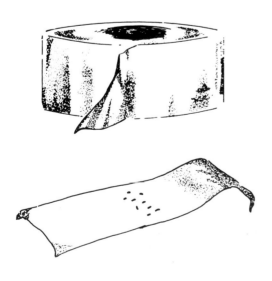

Vulvovaginitis may cause dysuria, vulval irritation, or a yellow stain on the pants, but the only abnormality to be seen may be a thin yellowish-grey vaginal discharge. The symptoms and even the results of a urine examination may be wrongly attributed to a urinary infection. Swabs (moistened with 0·9% sodium chloride solution) of the secretions are sent to the laboratory for microscopy and culture and the mother is taught how to collect a specimen for threadworm ova. When the child wakes in the morning, Sellotape is applied several times to the stretched perianal skin, and ova will adhere to it. Alternatively, ova can be collected from the perianal skin with a moist swab.

The only pathogens needing specific antimicrobial treatment are rare infections due to gonococci, monilia, or trichomonas. Antibiotic treatment of other organisms may result in fungal overgrowth causing iatrogenic disease. If no pathogens are detected the symptoms may be due to poor perineal hygiene and may resolve after twice daily baths. Detergents in poorly rinsed pants or "bubble baths" may cause a chemical vulvovaginitis. The remaining cases are usually related to a thin unstimulated vaginal mucosa. If the problem needs more than reassurance dienoestrol cream can be applied daily for three days and once a week for a month. This tiny dose thickens the mucosa. Longer treatment may cause withdrawal bleeding. A profuse purulent blood-streaked offensive discharge or symptoms which recur despite these measures are indications for examination under general anaesthesia to exclude a foreign body in the vagina.

Useful information

Some useful drugs

Children treated at home and most of those in hospital need oral drugs three times a day. They should be given before meals and the child need not be woken specially for the drug. Some preparations, particularly the penicillins, have an unpleasant taste and the medicine should not be mixed with food as the child may then hate both. Syrup, which is a sucrose solution that forms the base of most elixirs, may cause dental caries if it is given regularly for a long time. The concentration of the drug in the elixir should be high to provide a minimum volume. In difficult 1 to 3 year olds wrapping the child securely in a blanket may prevent spillage if only one adult is present to give the medicine. If a child will not accept a drug on a spoon the drug can be measured in a disposable syringe (with *no* needle) and squirted on to the child's tongue.

Aminophylline   3–5 mg/kg single intravenous dose given slowly
Amoxycillin   25–50 mg/kg/24 h orally
Ampicillin   50–100 mg/kg/24 h orally, intramuscularly,
   severe infections 300 mg/kg/24 h intravenously
Betamethasone   3 mg per dose intramuscularly or intravenously
Carbamazepine   10–20 mg/kg/24 h orally. Start with small dose
Ceftazidime   30–100 mg/kg/24 h intramuscularly or intravenously
Cephalexin   40–100 mg/kg/24 h orally
Chloral hydrate   30 mg/kg/24 h orally
Chlorpheniramine   1–2 mg per dose 3 times a day orally,
   intramuscularly, intravenously
Co-trimoxazole   6 mg/kg/24 h (as trimethoprim) orally
Diazepam   0·1–0·2 mg/kg orally or slowly intravenously
Dioctyl sodium sulphosuccinate   12·5 mg per dose 3 times
   daily orally
Erythromycin   50 mg/kg/24 h orally
Flucloxacillin   25–50 mg/kg/24 h orally, intramuscularly, or
   intravenously
Gentamicin   7 mg/kg/24 h intramuscularly or intravenously
Hyaluronidase   300 units per dose intramuscularly
Hydrocortisone   100 mg per dose intramuscularly or
   intravenously

Ipecacuanha paediatric emetic mixture   15 ml per dose
Methylcellulose 9% solution   5 ml per dose 3 times daily orally
Naloxone   0·01–0·02 mg/kg per dose intramuscularly or
   intravenously (can be repeated after 3 minutes)
Nitrofurantoin   2 mg/kg single dose daily by mouth as
   maintenance dose
Nystatin   100 000 units per dose (four hourly) orally *after* food
Paracetamol   75 mg/kg/24 h orally
Paraldehyde   0·2 ml/kg per dose intramuscularly
Penicillin   Benzylpenicillin   50 mg/kg/24 h intramuscularly
        severe infections 200 mg/kg/24 h intravenously
      Penicillin phenoxymethyl   50 mg/kg/24 h orally
Phenobarbitone   5 mg/kg/24 h orally or intramuscularly
Phenytoin   5 mg/kg/24 h orally or intramuscularly
Promethazine hydrochloride   1 mg/kg per dose orally or
   intramuscularly
Senna syrup (standardised)   2·5–5 ml per single daily dose
   orally
Sodium ironedetate   2·5–5·0 ml 3 times daily
Sodium valproate   20–30 mg/kg/24 h orally
Sulphafurazole   100 mg/kg/24 h orally
Trimeprazine tartrate   3 mg/kg per dose orally

Toys

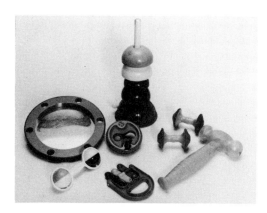

Toys appropriate for a child's development are useful in assessment but are also necessary to ensure that the child cooperates during the examination. Suitable toys for various ages include: press-up animals, elasticated collapse–return toys, snowstorms or shaking and turning toys, kaleidoscopes, miniature people, cars, crayons, telephones, rag dolls, crayons and paper, dolls' house and dolls' furniture, wooden puzzles, fitting plastic beakers, plastic rings on a pole. Suitable books include Ladybird first picture books 1–3 years, Mister Men 3–6 years. A glove puppet is also very useful for shy children, who will sometimes talk to a puppet but not to an adult. It can also be used to divert attention.

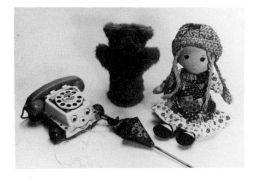

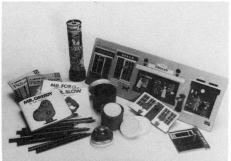

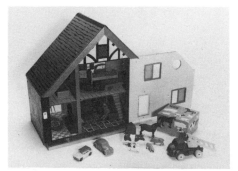

Guidance for parents of children with various illnesses or handicaps

Asthma—The Chest, Heart and Stroke Association, Tavistock House North, Tavistock Square, London WC1H 9JE (01-387 3012).
Leaflets: *Our child has asthma: some parents' questions answered; Breathing instructions for children.*

Blindness—The Royal National Institute for the Blind, 224 Great Portland Street, London W1N 6AA (01-388 1266).
Leaflet: *Changing all the time.*

Cerebral palsy and spasticity—The Spastics Society, 12 Park Crescent, London W1N 4EQ (01-636 5020).
Leaflets: *What is cerebral palsy?* And information pack for parents.

Coeliac disease—The Coeliac Society of the United Kingdom, PO Box 220, High Wickham, Bucks HP11 2HY (0494 37278), produces the *Coeliac Handbook* (£1·50), which incudes general, medical, and dietetic information on coeliac disease.

Cystic fibrosis—Cystic Fibrosis Trust, Alexandra House, 5 Blyth Road, Bromley BR1 3RS (01-464 7211).
Leaflet: *Cystic fibrosis.*

Deafness—National Deaf Children's Society, 45 Hereford Road, London W2 5AH (01-229 9272).
Leaflets: *You and your hearing impaired child; Testing the hearing of young children; Preparing your child for school; Some of the problems encountered by parents of hearing impaired children; Child development*; and other leaflets.

Royal National Institute for the Deaf, 105 Gower Street, London WC1E 6AH (01-387 8033).

Diabetes—British Diabetic Association, 10 Queen Anne Street, London W1N 0BD (01-323 1531).

Leaflets: *Children and adolescence: The diabetic at school; An introduction to diabetes.*

Disablement—Disabled Living Foundation, 380–4 Harrow Road, London W9 2HU (01-289 6111).
General information lists available.

Down syndrome—Down's Syndrome Association, 1st Floor, 12–13 Clapham Common South Side, London SW4 7AA (01-720 0008).
Leaflet: *You've had a Down's baby; Perhaps we can help*; and other information for parents.

Epilepsy—British Epilepsy Association, Anstey House, 40 Hanover Square, Leeds L53 1BE (0532 439393).
Leaflets: *Epilepsy: what to do; The schoolchild with epilepsy.*

Invalidity—Invalid Children's Aid Association, 126 Buckingham Palace Road, London SW1 W9SB (01-730 9891).

Mental handicap—Royal Society for Mentally Handicapped Children and Adults (MENCAP), 123 Golden Lane, London EC1Y 0RT (01-253 9433).
Leaflets: *A problem shared; Let's get it straight*; and other leaflets. Information sheets available.

Muscular dystrophy—Muscular Dystrophy Group of Great Britain and Northern Ireland, 35 Macaulay Road, London SW4 0QP (01-720 8055).

Physical handicap—Voluntary Council for Handicapped Children, 8 Wakley Street, London EC1V 7QE (01-278 9441).
Leaflet: *Help starts here: for parents of children with special needs* (50p). Lists of fact sheets available.

Spina bifida—Association for Spina Bifida and Hydrocephalus, 22 Upper Woburn Place, London WC1H 0EP (01-388 1382).
General leaflets available.

ACKNOWLEDGMENTS

I thank Blackwell Scientific Publications for allowing me to adapt liberally material that has appeared in *Accident and Emergency Paediatrics* and *Paediatric Therapeutics*. I also thank Richard Bowlby, Joanna Fairclough, Brian Pashley, Jeanette McKenzic, and Ann Shields of the department of medical illustration at Northwick Park Hospital for taking most of the photographs and Keith Bullock for several line drawings.

The remaining photographs were supplied as follows:

Sleep problems: the picture of Harry was reproduced from *Harry the Dirty Dog* by Gene Zion, illustrated by Margaret Bloy Graham, published by Bodley Head.

Tonsillitis and otitis media: illustration of eardrum and grommet from Valman B. *Keeping Babies and Children Healthy*. London: Martin Dunitz, 1985.

Bronchial asthma: the peak flow chart was reproduced from Godfrey S, *et al, British Journal of Diseases of the Chest* 1970;**64**:15.

Acute abdominal pain: inguinal hernia, Dr M Silverman and Dr Sheila McKenzie.

Chronic diarrhoea: jejunal biopsy specimens, Dr G Slavin.

Urinary tract infection: antibiotic sensitivity plate, Dr R F Williams; kidney scan, Dr Brendan Twomey.

Enuresis: the first illustration was adapted with permission from Dr M A Salmon and Spastic International Medical Publications from *Bladder Control and Enuresis* and the fifth by permission of Professor Roy Meadow. Mini-Drinite alarm and sensor by courtesy of Eastleigh Enuresis Alarms.

Systolic murmurs: the illustrations of ventricular septal defect and patent ductus arteriosus were adapted from *Essential Paediatrics* by David Hull and Derek I Johnstone, published by Churchill Livingstone.

Growth failure: the growth charts of 2–5 years and 0–19 years were adapted from those described by J M Tanner and R M Whitehouse in *Archives of Disease in Childhood* (1966 and 1975) and published by Castlemead Publications, Hertford (refs 28 and GDG 12A).

Infectious diseases: the illustrations were adapted from Krugman S, and Katz S L. *Infectious Diseases of Children*. 7th ed. St Louis: The C V Mosby Co, 1981.

Whooping cough: first graph, PHLS Communicable Disease Surveillance Centre; second graph, Dr N D Noah.

Recurrent headache: CT brain scan, Dr David Katz.

Accidents: illustrations 2, 4, 11, 12, and 13, RoSPA; 6, Dr R H Jackson; and 14 and 15, the Health Education Council.

Services for children: outpatient clinics and day care: a Nucleus children's nursing section, DHSS; growth chart from one described by D Gairdner and J Pearson in *Archives of Disease in Childhood* and published by Castlemead Publications, Hertford (Chart GPB).

I thank Dr H V L Finlay, who criticised most of the text, and Dr E M Brett, Professor S D M Court, Dr S R Goolamali, Mr H Gordon, Professor K S Holt, Dr R H Jackson, Dr D Morris, Dr R C Radley Smith, Mrs J Roberts, Dr R O Robinson, Dr E M Ross, Dr S M Samson, Dr J W G Smith, and Dr D A J Tyrrell, who each read parts of it.

For all photographs apart from those mentioned specifically above Dr H B Valman retains the copyright.

The drawing "The infant in the womb" by Leonardo da Vinci on the back cover is reproduced by gracious permission of Her Majesty the Queen.

Index

Index

126

Index